New Directions for Academic
Liaison Librarians

CHANDOS
INFORMATION PROFESSIONAL SERIES

Series Editor: Ruth Rikowski
(email: Rikowskigr@aol.com)

Chandos' new series of books are aimed at the busy information professional. They have been specially commissioned to provide the reader with an authoritative view of current thinking. They are designed to provide easy-to-read and (most importantly) practical coverage of topics that are of interest to librarians and other information professionals. If you would like a full listing of current and forthcoming titles, please visit www. chandospublishing.com or email wp@woodheadpublishing.com or telephone +44(0) 1223 499140.

New authors: we are always pleased to receive ideas for new titles; if you would like to write a book for Chandos, please contact Dr Glyn Jones on email gjones@chandospublishing.com or telephone number +44(0) 1993 848726.

Bulk orders: some organisations buy a number of copies of our books. If you are interested in doing this, we would be pleased to discuss a discount. Please contact on email wp@woodheadpublishing.com or telephone +44(0) 1223 499140.

New Directions for Academic Liaison Librarians

ALICE CRAWFORD

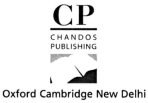

CHANDOS
PUBLISHING

Oxford Cambridge New Delhi

Chandos Publishing
Hexagon House
Avenue 4
Station Lane
Witney
Oxford OX28 4BN
UK
Tel: +44 (0) 1993 848726
Email: info@chandospublishing.com
www.chandospublishing.com
www.chandospublishingonline.com

Chandos Publishing is an imprint of Woodhead Publishing Limited

Woodhead Publishing Limited
80 High Street
Sawston
Cambridge CB22 3HJ
UK
Tel: +44(0) 1223 499140
Fax: +44(0) 1223 832819
www.woodheadpublishing.com

First published in 2012

ISBN: 978-1-84334-569-5 (print)

ISBN: 978-1-78063-304-6 (online)

© A. Crawford, 2012

British Library Cataloguing-in-Publication Data.
A catalogue record for this book is available from the British Library.

Typeset by RefineCatch Limited, Bungay, Suffolk.
Printed in the UK and USA.

Contents

Contents

Contents

Contents

List of abbreviations

AHRC	Arts and Humanities Research Council (UK)
ALA	American Library Association
ALISS	Association of Librarians and Information Professionals in the Social Sciences
APRIL	Australian Poetry Resource Library
ARC	Australian Research Council
ARL	Association of Research Libraries (US)
CABI	Centre for Agricultural Bioscience International
CAL	Copyright Agency Ltd (Australia)
CDL	California Digital Library
CIHR	Canadian Institutes of Health Research
CILIP	Chartered Institute of Library and Information Professionals
CVL	Community Virtual Library
DOI	Digital Object Identifier
DTD	Document Type Definition
EDFL	Educational Foundations and Leadership Graduate Program (George Fox University)
GFU	George Fox University, Portland, Oregon
HATII	Humanities Advanced Technology and Information Institute (University of Glasgow)
HE	Higher Education
HEO	Higher Education Officer
HINARI	Health InterNetwork Access to Research Initiative (WHO)
HUD	Heads Up Display

INASP	International Network for the Availability of Scientific Publications
ISSN	International Standard Serial Number
ISTE	International Society for Technology in Education
JISC	Joint Information Standards Committee (UK)
MALICO	Malawi Library and Information Consortium
METS	Metadata Encoding and Transmission Standard
MTPP	Mark Twain Papers & Project
MySQL	My (girl's name) Structured Query Language (Relational database management system)
NEH	National Endowment for the Humanities (USA)
NIH	National Institutes of Health (USA)
OA	Open Access
OBE	Order of the British Empire
OCLC	Online Computer Library Center, Inc.
OJS	Open Journal Systems
OSU	Ohio State University
PHP	Scripting language designed to produce dynamic web pages
RAE	Research Assessment Exercise (UK)
REF	Research for Excellence Framework (UK)
RIN	Research Information Network (UK)
RLSS	Research and Learning Support Services (University of Glasgow)
RLUK	Research Libraries UK
RPO	Research Policy Office (University of St Andrews)
SCONUL	Society of College, National & University Libraries (UK)
SDLC	Scottish Digital Libraries Consortium
SETIS	Sydney Electronic Text and Image Service
SUP	Sydney University Press

TCD	Trinity College, Dublin
TEI	Text Encoding Initiative
UBC	University of British Columbia
VLE	Virtual Learning Environment
VW	Virtual world
WHO	World Health Organization
XML	Extensible Markup Language
XSLT	Extensible Stylesheet Language Transformations
XTF	Extensible Text Framework

Acknowledgements

I am most grateful to the following people, who kindly agreed to be interviewed for this book, and who devoted time and energy to answering my questions, reading drafts and making valuable suggestions for improvement. I hope these case-studies provide a suitable showcase for their many impressive projects: Robin Ashford (Portland Center Library, George Fox University, Portland, Oregon); Susan Ashworth (University of Glasgow Library); Janet Aucock (University of St Andrews Library); Ross Coleman (University of Sydney Library); Vicki Cormie (University of St Andrews Library); Frances Gandy (Girton College Library, University of Cambridge); Dr Sharon K. Goetz (The Bancroft Library, University of California, Berkeley); Dr Catherine Mitchell (California Digital Library); Jackie Proven (University of St Andrews Library); Dr Stephen Rawles (Humanities Advanced Technology & Information Institute, University of Glasgow); and Dr Lisa Schiff (California Digital Library).

I am also extremely grateful to John MacColl, University Librarian and Director of Library Services at the University of St Andrews Library, whose help in introducing me to some of these interviewees, and in reading through my manuscript, has been invaluable.

Alice Crawford

About the author

Alice Crawford is Senior Academic Liaison Librarian for Arts and Divinity at the University of St Andrews Library. She has had a wide range of experience in libraries, having been librarian of a further education college as well as a subject librarian at Glasgow University Library, and worked in areas as varied and diverse as Special Collections, Engineering and Social Sciences. She has also enjoyed careers in university administration and teaching, having been a senior administrator at the University of Dundee and a teaching assistant in the University of St Andrews School of English.

She has published a research monograph, *Paradise Pursued: The Novels of Rose Macaulay* (Associated University Presses, 1995), based on her PhD thesis, as well as articles on librarianship. 'Getting back in: returning to libraries after a career break' appeared in *Impact*, Winter (2007): 73–5, and 'Academic liaison librarians: where do we stand?' appeared in *SCONUL Focus*, 45(2009): 34–7.

She has been a member of CILIP's University, College and Research Group's Scottish executive committee, and presented a paper, 'Academic liaison saves the world?', at the LILAC Conference 2008.

She holds MA (Hons) and PhD degrees from the University of Glasgow and an MA (Librarianship) degree from the University of Sheffield.

Introduction

Abstract: It is difficult to define what 'academic liaison' really means. The job has its roots in traditional subject librarianship, but more is now required. Liaison librarians need to be 'subject librarians plus'. The book will explore this 'plus' element and encourage liaison librarians to consider new possibilities. It will not attend to the well-worked area of information literacy teaching, but will offer case studies of other ventures. Case studies will show librarians setting up a medical library in Malawi, supporting the UK Research Assessment Exercise, teaching in virtual worlds, initiating digitisation and publishing projects, collaborating with academic colleagues to set up open access journals, managing outreach marketing activities, and project coordinating the design and delivery of a new library building. All will show liaison librarians maximising the potential of their new roles.

Key words: academic liaison, faculty liaison, librarianship, librarians, marketing, roles, subject librarians, subject librarianship, subject specialist.

What does academic liaison mean?

When I became an academic liaison librarian at the University of St Andrews Library in 2007, I remember grappling in dismay with the wide and disparate demands of my job

1

description. As liaison librarian for all the University's Arts and Divinity subjects, I was required to liaise with 19 academic departments; to develop information resources and services; to work with colleagues in the Collection Management team to ensure Library resources were exploited to maximum effect; to deliver information literacy and research skills programmes; to provide specialised information assistance and interventions; to develop liaison, communication and user training strategies through participation in university committees; to support the general enquiry service; to provide specialised subject support for all my subject areas; to engage in a full range of staff development activities, including presenting at conferences, writing articles and engaging in scholarly activities; to develop strategy and provide services relevant to the research and teaching needs of the university; to find new ways of communicating with customers and promoting Library resources; to assume cross-library responsibility for Official Publications and Reference Services . . . and to take on 'any other duties appropriate to the role'.

It was perhaps the rather desperate vagueness of that final 'any other duties' clause which confirmed for me the uncertainty and lack of clarity with which the writers of the job specification had approached the task. What does 'academic liaison' *mean*? What is an academic liaison librarian supposed to do? My four years in post have involved me in an ongoing effort to answer that question, and have in many ways simply confirmed the difficulties. With its requirements of 'specialised information assistance' and 'specialised subject support', the job has its roots in good old-fashioned subject librarianship. Yet the specification does muddle its way towards recognising that more is required of the new breed of subject/liaison librarian. Information literacy teaching is a clear and prominent requirement, but less clearly defined are the injunctions to 'find new ways of communicating with customers' and to 'develop strategy and provide services relevant to research and teaching needs'. What could these new ways of communicating be? What services *are* relevant to a university's research and teaching needs? There is an awareness in this job description that the new liaison librarian needs to be the old subject librarian PLUS – but what this PLUS element should constitute is frustratingly, if understandably, undefined.

It is with the possibilities of this PLUS element that *New Directions for Academic Liaison Librarians* is concerned. The book will aim to encourage liaison librarians to think beyond the traditional realms of academic librarianship to explore new possibilities for their role. It will for the most part bypass the field of information literacy teaching to showcase the many other areas in which academic liaison librarians can engage in collaborative projects with academic staff. It will show the full potential of the liaison role and emphasise the need for flexibility, imagination and initiative in those who hold these posts. It will give concrete and interesting examples of academic liaison in practice, countering – I hope – the idea that 'liaison' is simply a question of constant and patient attendance at academic drinks parties to soak up information, or even just gossip, which will help librarians discover what their readers need. Liaison can mean going out to Malawi to help university administrators and academics set up a medical library for a community with the poorest patient–doctor ratio in the world. It can mean working with academics and poets to create a national poetry database, or establishing a viable publishing business from a library's manuscript holdings. It can mean using traditional 'librarianly' skills in a new way to ensure the bibliographic quality of a university's submission to the REF or RAE, or helping to re-establish a library's reputation for scholarship by launching an ambitious programme of public lectures. This book aims not only to reassure liaison librarians of the value of their role, but also to inspire them with ideas for its potential. Liaison librarianship is, as a colleague recently remarked, an area of our profession which is rather confused about its future. This book hopes to help by showing that there is a useful way forward for those working in this area, but that it will involve the hard work of breaking new ground.

From subject librarian to academic liaison?

If liaison librarianship is currently dealing with the problems of its uncertain future, it can at least be said that it emerged from a secure past. The 'subject librarian' role from which it grew was for many years the safe and unchallenged backbone of UK and US academic library structures. Fred J. Hay produces a useful consideration of 'The Subject Specialist in the Academic Library' (1990), his insights helpfully expanded and updated later in the decade by J.V. Martin in his 'Subject Specialization in British University Libraries' (1996).[1] Derek Law's chapter on 'The Organization of Collection Management in Academic Libraries' (1999) provides further pertinent contributions to the subject, while Richard Gaston offers the most comprehensive overview (2001) of writing in this area, identifying models of subject librarianship in different countries for comparison with the UK role, and considering how the role has been defined before and after the Follett report of 1993.[2] It is in Stephen Pinfold's (2001) article, however, that the first sense of real anxiety about the role emerges, as he summarises the traditional responsibilities of the subject librarian (enquiry work, selection of material and management of budgets, cataloguing and classification, collection management, user education, production of guides and publicity) and moves on to consider those of the changing role (more liaison with users, advocacy of the collections, enquiries assisted by new technology, working with technical staff, selection of e-resources, information skills training, organising the information landscape, involvement in educational technology, team working, and project working).[3] Here for the first time we find an attempt being made to define what liaison might mean – there must be, says Pinfold, 'more emphasis on "getting out there" rather than expecting users to come to the library', and on doing everything possible to connect the subject librarian to the user more closely, before he begins to feel, erroneously of course, that he may be able to find all relevant information himself without the help of a library intermediary. In 'Dinosaur or Dynamo? The Future for the Subject Specialist Reference Librarian', John Rodwell (2001) proposes an intelligent and passionate defence of traditional subject specialist skills, concluding,

> If 'disintermediation' is a threat to librarians, it is perhaps the generalist who is in danger of going the way of the dinosaur. The subject specialist may well be the dynamo in any organisation for which information is crucial.[4]

The fullest treatment of the subject librarian role is provided by Penny Dale, Matt Holland and Marian Matthews in their book, *Subject Librarians: Engaging with the Learning and Teaching Environment* (2006).[5] Discussions of the role now assume that the metamorphosis of the Subject Librarian into Faculty Liaison Librarian, Academic Liaison Librarian or Faculty Support Librarian is complete, and that the new skill sets of these post-holders are unchallenged – they need to be teachers and communicators, fast learners, with vision and advanced technical and IT skills and an ability to build teams, manage projects and be aware of the varying needs of their different constituencies (undergraduates, researchers, international students, asynchronous learners, and so on). Dale et al. see the new subject librarian as a driver for change in an electronic library environment, and as

> uniquely placed to develop the role of knowledge broker, working with students and academics to consolidate and enhance their contributions to learning and teaching. The need to collaborate and find new ways of working with faculty and students is one of the themes of [their] book.
>
> (2006, p. 191)

The theme is taken up again most recently by Linden Fairbairn and John Rodwell in their (2008) article, 'Dangerous liaisons? Defining the faculty liaison service model, its effectiveness and sustainability', which examines variations in the definitions of the role, the expectations of the post-holders, their managers and clients, and the impact of environmental factors.[6] It shows how the emerging role is characterised by a more outward-looking perspective and complexity, with an emphasis on strong involvement and partnership with academic staff and direct engagement with the university's teaching and research programmes.

Antony Brewerton's (2009) initiative in producing a 'Subject Librarian' issue of *SCONUL Focus* has usefully turned the spotlight on the current situation in this area of the profession, and provided an interesting cross-section of activities across the sector.[7] In a collection of some 40 articles, liaison librarians across the UK describe here how they have adapted to the changing requirements of their jobs, acquiring new teaching and IT skills, and developing information literacy modules which they work hard to have embedded in timetabled academic courses. The impression given is of a lively, active, professional community, wholeheartedly embracing change and enjoying the opportunities offered. In his interesting editorial introduction to the issue, Brewerton reports that he had recently put out a request on library lists for colleagues to send him copies of subject librarian job descriptions, and had been impressed by the enthusiastic response. Replies had been received from 33 institutions, and details of 62 posts had been submitted. Interestingly, nearly all had contained the 'traditional' requirements of the subject librarian role – liaison with the academic community, collection management and development, budget management, information skills training, enquiry support, production of library guides, web-pages, and so on. Most, too, had been concerned predominantly with teaching and learning support. There had, however, been an encouraging sense in many of the job descriptions of the 'opening out' of the liaison librarian's portfolio to include other areas. Some had asked for engagement with RAE/REF support, with e-learning activities, staff management, project work and marketing. In general, there had been an awareness of new possibilities on the horizon, and a receptiveness to the opportunities that change might bring – 'Change looks to be a constant in many of the posts reviewed,' Brewerton concludes.

Subject librarians 'plus'

It is with this 'opening out' of the liaison librarian's portfolio in the face of change that this book is concerned. It will not be attending to the well-worked area of information literacy teaching, about which much has already been written, but will be pushing out into territory less known. It will describe the experiences of librarians who have been involved in collaborative projects with academics which have allowed their professional skills to be displayed and used at levels not previously recognised. Case studies will show librarians supporting the RAE, initiating major digitisation and publishing ventures, designing new library buildings, teaching in virtual worlds with academic colleagues, collaborating with faculty to set up open access journals, managing outreach and marketing activities, and taking library management skills to the developing world. The aim will be to display the full potential of the new liaison librarian's support role.

The urgency with which this support role needs to be claimed is apparent in OCLC's recent *Support for the Research Process: An Academic Library Manifesto* (2009), in which Chris Bourg, Ross Coleman and Ricky Erway call academic libraries to action if they are to continue to play a central role in the field of scholarly research and publishing.[8] The imperatives are, they say, to study the ever-changing work patterns and needs of researchers, to design flexible new services around those parts of the research process that cause researchers the most frustration and difficulty, to embed library content, services and staff within researchers' regular workflows, to embrace the role of expert information navigators and redefine reference as research consultation instead of fact-finding. Academic libraries must also, they say, embrace opportunities to focus on unique, core services and resources, and find ways of demonstrating to university administrators and auditors the value to scholarship of library services and resources. They must, too, engage researchers in the identification of primary research data sets that merit long-term preservation and access, and offer alternative scholarly publishing and dissemination platforms which are integrated with appropriate repositories and preservation services.

Overview of the book

New Directions for Academic Liaison Librarians offers case studies in which all these imperatives are addressed. In Chapter 1, Vicki Cormie at St Andrews has used her knowledge of medical library resources to contribute significantly to the redevelopment, restocking and streamlining of library procedures at the Malawi College of Medicine. In Chapter 2, Susan Ashworth describes how her team at Glasgow University Library have impressed on university administrators the value of their bibliographic checking skills to the complex RAE submission process. Chapter 3 describes how Robin Ashford has worked enthusiastically with academic colleagues to acclimatize students at George Fox University to the challenging but attractive virtual world of Second Life. In Chapter 4, in the three case studies presented there, we learn how Ross Coleman has revived the Sydney University Press imprint, and worked with poets and academic colleagues to create and copyright clear digital material for the Australian Poetry Library database. We also discover how Stephen Rawles at the University of Glasgow has brought both his scholarly and librarianly skills to the creation of the impressive Glasgow Emblem Digitisation Project, and, finally, how Catherine Mitchell's staff at the California Digital Library have established their eScholarship initiative to publish and disseminate materials required by the scholarly community, and to provide digital access to unique resources such as the Mark Twain Papers.

Chapter 5 shows how Repository Support Officer Jackie Proven at the University of St Andrews Library has used the opportunities provided by the OJS (Open Journal Systems) platform to have useful conversations with faculty and postgraduate students about shaping their proposed open access journals, as well as about Open Access, repositories and e-scholarship generally.

At the University of St Andrews Library I have found valuable new ways of communicating with the Library's town and gown communities through the varied activities of a Friends of the Library group, and this is the case study presented in Chapter 6.

Finally, in Chapter 7, Frances Gandy at Girton College, Cambridge, has proved to her College Executive that a librarian's specialist knowledge of what a library building must be designed to do has enabled her to make a unique and essential contribution to fundraising initiatives for a new one.

Karen Williams and Janice Jaguscewski's forthcoming report, *Transforming Liaison Roles*, in the ARL's *New Roles for New Times* series promises further discussion of ways in which academic libraries are currently grappling to redefine the new liaison role.[9] A broadened definition of liaison librarian roles is, as Williams says, key:

> Liaisons are challenged to become more outwardly focused, striving to understand the needs and changing practices of scholars and students in order to shape future directions. Building strong relationships with faculty and other campus professionals, and establishing collaborative partnerships within and across institutions will be necessary building blocks to our success.

Here, then, are some true stories in which liaison librarians have maximised the potential of their newly broadened role-definitions, become more outwardly focused, built strong relationships with faculty, and established a variety of collaborative partnerships in a range of institutions. They are – surely – success stories about the continuing value of the librarian's role. I hope they inspire!

Notes

1. Fred J. Hay, 'The subject specialist in the academic library: a review article', *The Journal of Academic Librarianship*, 16(1) (1990): 11–17. J.V. Martin, 'Subject specialization in British university libraries: a second survey', *Journal of Librarianship and Information Science*, 28(3) (1996): 159–69.
2. Derek Law, 'The organization of collection management in academic libraries', in Clare Jenkins and Mary Morley (eds), *Collection Management in Academic Libraries*, 2nd edn (Aldershot: Gower, 1999): 15–37. Richard Gaston, 'The changing role of the subject librarian, with a particular focus on UK developments, examined through a review of the literature', *New Review of Academic Librarianship*, 7(1) (2001): 19–36.
3. Stephen Pinfield, 'The changing role of subject librarians in academic libraries', *Journal of Librarianship and Information Science*, 33(1) (2001): 32–8.
4. John Rodwell, 'Dinosaur or dynamo? The future for the subject specialist reference librarian', *New Library World*, 102(1/2) (2001): 48–52.
5. Penny Dale, Matt Holland and Marian Matthews, *Subject Librarians: Engaging with the Learning and Teaching Environment* (Aldershot: Ashgate, 2006).
6. Linden Fairbairn and John Rodwell, 'Dangerous liaisons? Defining the faculty liaison librarian service model, its effectiveness and sustainability', *Library Management*, 29(1/2) (2008): 116–24. DOI: 10.1108/01435120810844694.
7. Antony Brewerton, The Subject Librarian, Special Issue, *SCONUL Focus* (45) (2009): 3–4.
8. Chris Bourg, Ross Coleman and Ricky Erway, *Support for the Research Process: an Academic Library Manifesto. Report Produced by OCLC Research* (2009). Available at: *http://www.oclc.org/research/publications/library/2009/2009-07.pdf*.
9. Karen Williams and Janice Jaguscewski, *Transforming Liaison Roles*. Forthcoming report in the ARL's *New Roles for New Times* Series. Available at: *http://www.arl.org/rtl/plan/nrnt/nrntliaison.shtml*.

Liaison in the wider world: a medical librarian in Malawi

Abstract: Vicki Cormie, liaison librarian at St Andrews University, joined a team of university academic and administrative staff involved in a long-term project to deliver medical education in Malawi. Her role was to ensure that students had adequate access to print and electronic resources at the library of the Malawian College of Medicine, in Blantyre. Problems of unreliable internet access, the lack of professional library staff, and uncatalogued, out-of-date stock were encountered and solutions to these problems were discussed. The experience offered rich opportunities for liaison with university administration and IT colleagues, as well as with Malawian library staff. Vicki returned exhilarated by the experience, pleased to have had her role valorised and to have felt appreciated as a respected and integral member of the team, with a clear part to play.

Key words: academic liaison, case study, faculty liaison, liaison, librarians, librarianship, library, Malawi, medical librarianship, Third World.

Background to the project

'I never thought when I became a librarian that it was a job where you got to fly off and visit exciting places!' wrote Vicki Cormie in the St Andrews University Library newsletter the week before she set out to share her professional skills with library staff in the College of Medicine at the University of Malawi, in Africa.

As Senior Academic Liaison Librarian for Science and Medicine, Vicki was delighted to be asked to join a team of St Andrews academic and administrative staff involved in a long-term project to develop support for the delivery of medical education in Malawi. Funded by the Scottish Government's Malawi Development Programme, which had allocated £252,000 over three years, the scheme built on a long-standing relationship between the University of St Andrews and the Malawian College of Medicine, and aimed to increase healthcare provision in the area by training more doctors. The Malawian College of Medicine was founded in 1991 on the model of medical training provided at St Andrews, and this historical connection, coupled with the fact that St Andrews' Bute Medical School had just completed an expansion-based curriculum reform of the same kind as that required by the Malawians, led to a Memorandum of Understanding being signed by the two institutions in March 2008. It was agreed that the two institutions should collaborate over curriculum reform, and work together to support that reform through an improved infrastructure of IT and other research resources.

Offers of assistance from the Scottish team were particularly timely, arriving as they did at a point of severe crisis in Malawi's healthcare provision. With just one doctor per 200,000 people – the lowest ratio in the world – the country's need was obvious and acute. The principal goal of the St Andrews project was therefore to increase the number of doctors being trained per year from 16 to 100, and to educate them more efficiently by introducing a more up-to-date curriculum. Key to this would be the delivery of substantial quantities of teaching via a virtual learning environment

(VLE), enabling students to develop independent learning skills while cutting down on staff contact hours and on time spent marking. Vicki was recognised as a key member of the team; her skills were seen to be clearly essential in ensuring that, once the VLE was up and running, there would be efficient access to appropriate library resources.

Initial impressions

Flying out in October 2008, the four academics in the group set to work with their Malawian colleagues to help restructure the medical curriculum. Drawing on their own recent experience of curriculum overhaul, they facilitated the development of a new series of modules which covered all the basic and clinical skills necessary for the training of a greatly increased number of students, while rationalising and streamlining the use of lecturing staff time, reducing the number of lectures by half and the number of examinations to be passed from 27 to one. The emphasis in these new modules was to be on introducing the new concept of self-directed learning to the Malawian students, with the aim of producing doctors with the enhanced critical thinking skills which would emerge from this more problem-based learning. Phenomenal progress was made, and by the end of their visit the team had redesigned and re-written the first-year curriculum, and produced concrete plans for future years.

Vicki was alert from the start to the academic liaison potential of being part of a multi-disciplinary team. She joined the academic group at the beginning of November along with staff from Business Improvements, IT Services and the Principal's Office. While the IT staff concentrated on installing a significant number of PCs and setting up an intranet, and the Registry staff worked on developing the online student record system which would make the VLE functional, Vicki explored with the librarian and his team the many problems attendant on attempting to provide swift, reliable access to electronic resources in a country where both bandwidth and sheer numbers of PCs via which to connect to it were cripplingly limited. It was clear that all elements of the team were interdependent. The curriculum could not be developed without the academics, or delivered without technical and administrative input from IT Services and Business Improvements, while Vicki's knowledge of library resources was crucially relevant to both. They all had to work together, contributing their separate areas of expertise and consulting constantly with one another as they moved towards a common goal.

Vicki wrote in her blog,[1] shortly after her arrival:

> One of the first things that I have discovered since getting here is that the internet is very dodgy everywhere. I really understand now about the problems that people have here with internet bandwidth . . . As well as poor connectivity, there are frequent power cuts, both planned as part of a nationwide energy-saving programme and more haphazard. I thought in my innocence that the candle in the room was a nice decorative touch. At the hotel, the wifi seems to go down for a day or two after each power cut too, which is a real pain.

Her blog records her vivid first impressions of this hot, bright world which was to be the scene of her academic liaison activities for some two weeks.

> Flying into the airport at Blantyre was a bit like arriving at a cricket pavilion. The viewing platforms were fully

packed with families presumably not all waiting for people to come in, but rather enjoying the spectacle. The heat was the first thing that hit us coming out of the plane . . .

We sense her excitement as she tunes in to the new sights, sounds and smells of the place:

I wasn't expecting so many trees, and certainly not so many in colour. Vivid pinks and oranges (some sort of jacaranda I think) and bougainvillea . . . The sounds are an amazing mixture. In the evening you can sit outside and hear the call to prayer, crickets and grasshoppers, distant party-goers all at the same time. The smells are of wood smoke which permeates everywhere after dark, eucalyptus and warm earth.

Working with the library

However, her engagement with the important project in hand was always at the forefront of her mind. To her surprise, she found the College library rather better provisioned than she had expected. Established in 1990, it stocked, according to its website (last updated in 2006), some 20,000 book volumes, 15,600 bound periodicals and 42 current periodical titles. It had good study spaces, was well used by the medical students, and reminded her, on the whole, of a UK nursing library in which she had worked some ten years previously. A growing range of electronic resources supplemented the print ones, made available by means of financial help from such organisations as INASP, MALICO and WHO.[2] Databases included African Journals Online, Blackwell Synergy, Cambridge University Press, Emerald, HINARI,

Oxford Reference Online, Wiley Interscience, Pubmed and CAB Abstracts. On closer inspection, however, difficulties became apparent. There were only two professionally qualified members of staff, of whom one was on maternity leave at the time of Vicki's visit. Stock was out of date in some areas, and uncatalogued donations had accumulated on the shelves. While there was access in theory to a surprisingly large number of scientific e-journals (often donated freely or cheaply by publishers to universities in developing countries), in practice painfully slow internet connections and poor search facilities meant that they were not much used. Technically available, they were unindexed and unsearchable. Depressingly, too, it was clear that it would be some time before bandwidth would be expanded to improve connection speeds. In addition, Vicki realised that, fundamentally, the Library was itself being used in a very different way from what she was used to in the UK – holding multiple (i.e. dozens of!) copies of course texts, it served in effect as a book bank rather than a library, providing textbooks for every student on a course. Students were not familiar with the concept of browsing to find books on particular topics, and the catalogue was in many ways redundant. Unsupported by the IT provider from which it had been bought, it was frequently simply not switched on – and students did not, in any case, need it to locate items on the 'book bank' shelves. With the introduction of more problem-based learning and critical thinking skills into the medical curriculum, Vicki realised it was likely to be only a matter of time before students would need to be educated in new ways of searching and acquiring information from the library's stock.

She spent the first few days observing what was going on, noting the Library's strengths and weaknesses, and adjusting to the situation on the ground, which proved rather different from what she had expected. She now had insight into what it is like to be on the receiving end of well-meaning charity initiatives. Foreign aid had ensured that an impressive number of volumes had reached the library, but they were not necessarily the ones the students wanted or the ones that their courses demanded. Staff had little time to process donations, and inadequate cataloguing and classification made these new resources often difficult to locate. Similar aid initiatives had paid for a large, new library building, but not for fitting it out – there was no money for bookshelves, photocopiers or an automated circulation system. The result, it seemed to Vicki, was a library which, despite myriad good intentions, had not yet evolved fully into twenty-first-century mode. Her efforts, therefore, became very much focused on providing what immediate practical solutions she could.

An initial area in which library help could be offered was in attempting to manage the many electronic journals, listing them and making them searchable. Vicki advised on the availability of the open source serials management system, CUFTS, which would provide the necessary functionality.[3] On her return to the UK, she would be able to provide training on how to set this up, and plans to move forward with this when she has access to the library server in Malawi – a more complicated procedure than she had initially anticipated!

Arrangements were also put in train for a batch of new computers and a new server, purchased with funding from the Scottish Parliament, to be sent out to the library. Money was made available, too, to purchase extra bandwidth for the library, though this was recognised as merely a temporary solution. IT staff on the team advised on the university's web pages, introducing some technical adjustments which would improve the speed of response.

The team also realised the importance in the longer term of developing students' information skills, and worked hard to devise relevant information skills modules for all curriculum years, with the exception of the pre-medical year, which presented particular problems. Topics covered were the usual ones of how to recognise and use appropriate databases, how to conduct a literature search, how to define search terms, how to limit or expand sets of references retrieved, and how to assess the quality of web-based material. In due course, Vicki hoped, library staff would take over from IT and academic staff in delivering the content of these modules, and would assume a more proactive guidance role. Meantime, however, she felt that their priorities ought to be developing the more essential library processes – establishing a robust and usable online catalogue and introducing a dependable serials management system.

Networking and liaison

Vicki has definitely found the experience enriching and rewarding at many levels. One of her colleagues on the trip was the library representative for Medicine, and the sense of shared adventure here undoubtedly helped strengthen an already good professional relationship. The group worked consistently well as a team of equal members. Daily meetings morning and evening allowed exchange of information and important catch-up to take place. Opportunities were offered for gaining insight into what each side did, and the process of working together towards a common achievable goal was satisfying. Library, administrative and IT staff sat in on many of the academics' discussions on the curriculum, and there was a real sense of each section contributing to the work of the others. The presence of senior figures from the Malawi

University executive valorised the project and reassured team members that their input was worthwhile, and appreciated by the wider academic community. The Library in particular was pleased to have been made an integral part of the project. The team's recognition of Vicki's contribution to the venture provided morale-boosting confirmation that librarians still have much to offer in an age where 'everyone's a librarian now'.

Post-project activities

Follow-up to the visit has been consistently positive and productive. After a subsequent trip by the team to Malawi in November 2009, plans are now underway to progress a second, separate, non-governmental, project which will provide developmental aid for the community of Muona in the south of the country. A team from the University of St Andrews Students' Association has taken over this project and is busily engaged in fundraising efforts which aim to strengthen relationships between the student and school communities in both countries. As an active member of this team, Vicki is pleased to be continuing her Malawi connection, and is happy to be helping to raise the project's profile.

In general, Vicki has had a sense of expanding her horizons. She warmed to the people she met. 'The people have exceeded any expectation of the friendliness I was told about,' she writes in her blog. 'You can see why Malawi is known as the warm heart of Africa. Everywhere people are so genuinely kind and welcoming and a smile is always met back warmly.' Five-hour journeys over dried-up river beds in the back of a van with less than luxurious sideways seats brought the wonderful rewards of sights and sounds in Liwonde National

Park which will stay with her always – hundreds of elephants, hippos, crocodiles, warthogs, buffalo, baboons and antelopes, plus eagles, kingfishers and unidentifiable exotic birds which dazzled the keen photographer with their 'electric greens and blues and bright yellow'.

The experience has left her with an acute awareness of Western material advantages, and opened her eyes to the different African way of life, where a sense of community is dominant, but where extreme poverty is endemic, pervasive and distressing. She was conscious always on both her visits of the missing generations, lost to disease, and of her own sense of helplessness before the vastness and intractability of the problem. The visitor's ability to 'switch off' to the difficulty on return to the West was, she found, guilt-inducing but necessary. Interestingly, the project has also brought her into contact with a surprising number of other people in the library world who are working in similar areas; blogging and talking about her experiences at conferences has allowed her to meet a Western community enthusiastic about trying to provide support for fellow library workers in the developing world.

Most memorable, however, will be her pictures of the 'real view of Malawian life' the adventure afforded her – the smiling people, the waving children, the little boys playing in front of their house as the van drove past. She has returned having met people who value learning, who suffer much to obtain it, who struggle to connect with books both print and electronic, and who recognise that the knowledge contained within them is hard-won but priceless. She has visited a land where libraries and learning are appreciated, and has the ongoing satisfaction of knowing that the contributions she and her team colleagues have made have been worthwhile. The professional liaisons which have coalesced in this project have made a difference.

Lessons learned for similar projects

Vicki found it important to approach her project in an open-minded way. Taking her lead from other members of the team who have worked in the area previously, she has learned not to impose 'textbook' solutions on situations, but to watch and wait, observing what people really require and working with them gradually to reach outcomes which will be workable-with in the long term. She found a flexible, open-minded approach to be best and has learned to draw efficiently on the many skills of the team, making her own contribution in an equitable and enriching way. If others have worked in the field already, it is sensible to call on that ready-developed expertise rather than to start from scratch to try to acquire it. Involvement in this project has allowed Vicki to observe the dynamics of team-working and to experiment with and optimise her own possible roles. She has enjoyed the 'give and take' of the team, and offers some psychological insights into the workings of the group, noting, for example, that people generally like being seen to be contributing to a good cause, and are gratified by that involvement. 'No man is an island' and any team's achievement is necessarily the result of its members' efficient and focused liaison with one another.

Vicki's advice for those considering embarking on a similar project:

- Don't go with preconceived ideas about what to expect – the reality is likely to be quite different. Be open to the experience.

- Use the resources of established experts in the field rather than trying to operate alone and 'reinvent the wheel'. Bodies such as INASP can provide advice and practical help in projects like this.

- Work with the team, and use the different specialisms of all team members and of staff in your home institution. People are usually glad to help, and you shouldn't feel that you have sole responsibility for the project's delivery.

Notes

1. Vicki's adventures in Malawi: available at: *http://vickimalawi. blogspot.com/*.
2. INASP: International Network for the Availability of Scientific Publications; MALICO: Malawi Library and Information Consortium; WHO: World Health Organization.
3. CUFTS Open Source Serials Management: available at: *http:// researcher.sfu.ca/cufts*.

2

Liaison and bibliometric support: the UK Research Assessment Exercise

Abstract: A number of liaison librarians were closely engaged with the UK's Research Assessment Exercise (RAE) in 2008 and found this an important new direction in which to develop. Susan Ashworth had responsibility for the team within Research and Learning Support Services at the University of Glasgow Library, which worked on the Glasgow University submission and had the job of checking for accuracy the outputs of all research-active academic staff. She describes the stresses and strains of the exercise, as well as its satisfactions, and suggests that liaison and other librarians can have a significant role to play, not only in ensuring the accuracy of the bibliographic input but also in resolving the many queries and difficulties which arise during the RAE process.

Key words: academic liaison, bibliometrics, faculty liaison, institutional repositories, Key Perspectives, liaison, librarians, librarianship, RAE, REF, Research Assessment Exercise, Research for Excellence Framework, University of Glasgow Library.

Background to the project: what is the RAE?

'It has been suggested that best practice would be for the library to have a subject or liaison librarian for every department in an institution, so they really come to understand the research outputs and can work with researchers to provide a range of information or data-related services – not only to curate outputs, but also to advise them on matters central to research assessment such as where to publish, research impact and bibliometrics.' So write the authors of OCLC's 2009 study of the role of libraries in the research assessment process, their insight reflecting an encouraging grasp of the potential available to the new-breed liaison librarian who wishes to move in the new direction offered by involvement in the UK Research Assessment Exercise – now enjoying the updated nomenclature of the Research Excellence Framework.[1]

Prepared by Key Perspectives Ltd, the report offers a useful synopsis of how research assessment processes have developed in the UK as well as in the Netherlands, Ireland, Denmark and Australia. The USA is not included in the study as it has no national research assessment regime, and the different funding environment there makes comparison with the five other countries examined impossible. The UK is distinctive in the closeness with which it ties its assessment process to funding, using the RAE results to determine the distribution of Quality Related (QR) research funds to universities. (Funding from the Research Councils, it should be noted, is administered separately.) There have been six national research assessment exercises in the UK since 1986, the most recent one in 2008 involving the assessment of 2344 submissions from 159 Higher Education institutions. The 2008 RAE differed from its predecessors in that results were published as a quality profile rather than using a fixed scale, and assessment was done within a two-tier panel structure. Over 1000 people, chosen for their subject expertise, formed the assessment panels, their aim being to apply quality classifications according to a five-point scale ranging from Unclassified (quality which falls below the standard of nationally recognised work) to 4* (quality which is world-leading in terms of originality, significance and rigour). The closing date for submissions to the next UK research assessment exercise – the Research Excellence Framework, or REF – is now 29 November 2013, and the signs are that it intends to make greater use of 'quantitative indicators' and to take into account the impact of research on the economy, society and public policy.

In general, the report finds, the RAE is seen to have achieved its goals. Researchers see the point of it and agree that it can improve individuals' performances and make them more accountable. It provides a means of benchmarking institutions, and has been accepted as authoritative by most academics because it is based on peer review. Yet compliance with the scheme represents significant costs in terms of time, bureaucracy and finance. Being so explicitly tied to funding makes engagement in the process a heavy administrative burden for every institution. Researchers are put under great pressure to make the strongest possible contribution to their department's submission, and in some ways the exercise can result in distorting the way researchers work. The new emphasis on conducting externally funded research, for example, seems to encourage academics to focus on writing grant proposals rather than writing books. The system generates competing lists of winners and losers, and, while departments which perform well enjoy prestige and additional funding, those which receive lower rankings are caught in a downward spiral of low morale and lack of funding.

Library contribution to the RAE: the Glasgow University experience

Though comparatively little has been written about liaison librarians' contribution to the RAE, it is clear that many in the UK have in fact been closely engaged in the process leading up to the 2008 submission, and continue to have input both in the 'aftermath' stage and in the 'regrouping and preparation' stage of the next round.[2] Susan Ashworth of the University of Glasgow provides helpful insight into the RAE experiences of staff in her own library, and confirms that several of the subject librarians there, particularly in the Arts and Social Sciences, made a significant contribution.[3] She is clear that this is an important role for subject/liaison librarians to move into:

> At Glasgow, we have a subject-based liaison-led organisational structure for our subject librarians, which, especially on the science side, is a model we are slowly revising. The demand for traditional subject librarian support in many science subjects has been diminishing as desk-top access to information provision has dramatically improved. Very few academic staff in science subjects use the physical library or seek mediation with regard to searching for information (with the exception of medicine), but there is increasing demand for other services such as bibliographic software packages; institutional repository services; plagiarism-detection software; bibliometrics; the management of publications data; and curation and preservation of

research outputs, potentially including research data. These are all areas where subject librarians are taking a lead at the University of Glasgow.[4]

Asked to administer the RA2 (Research Outputs) element of Glasgow's 2008 RAE submission, staff at her library were given the perfect opportunity to demonstrate their dependability and skill in the management of publications data. As Assistant Director for Research and Learning Support Services, Susan herself had overall responsibility for the Library contribution to the project, and worked closely with the Deputy Head of the Library's IT Unit and the administrator for RLSS, who together formed the core of staff working on the submission. RAE 'champions' were appointed for each Unit of Assessment, and subject librarians liaised with these single points of contact in the Departments to resolve problems or queries in person. This system worked well, allowing library staff to cement relationships with academics, and to gain increased insight into the research specialisms of each area.

At the university level, the wider administration of the submission was the responsibility of the Research Planning and Strategy Committee (RPSC), which devolved the detail of the work to an RAE Administrators' Group which included staff from the Library. Following the RAE, the Research Planning and Strategy Committee set up a Bibliometrics Working Party, and Susan represented the Library on this group, along with a member of staff from Research and Enterprise and a senior academic from each of the university's three academic territories. It was the job of the Working Party to monitor the use of bibliometrics and citation data to ensure that the university was prepared for any move toward a greater use of metrics, and, while this working group has now folded, the university has now created a REF Working Party, with Library representation, which keeps a close eye on developments affecting the dynamics of the next assessment submission and has responsibility, among other things, for the university's strategy in relation to bibliometrics.

Process details

It was the job of the Library's RA2 team to check for accuracy the research outputs of all members of staff being submitted for the RAE (each person being required to select their 'top 4' for the time period of 1 January 2001 – 31 December 2007), and ensure that access was available, either online or in print copy, to the full text of each item.[5] Over 5000 items were sourced, checked and entered into the RAE database. A wide range of inconsistencies were encountered. Partial or incomplete references meant that DOIs (Digital Object Identifiers) were not picked up automatically by the system and so had to be searched for in the Library's e-journals or bibliographic databases. Exact dates of publication had to be found for each journal article, a surprisingly difficult task when there was no DOI available, since print and online dates could sometimes vary significantly. ISSNs threw up many problems of verification, as did the tracking down of articles in journals to which the Library did not subscribe. For the latter, staff were often obliged to liaise with departmental administrators or academics themselves to obtain personal copies which could be scanned to create pdf files and sent as a separate submission on CD to the RAE. Occasionally an electronic copy had to be bought from a publisher, if no other version was available. Print copies of books were meticulously marshalled, labelled, listed and boxed before being finally sent on their way by road to RAE headquarters. Towards the end, problems of items still pending publication caused particular concern, and the team liaised constantly with author and publisher about expected publication dates for these as the RAE deadline loomed.

Opportunities for the library

A challenging exercise throughout, the project allowed the team to display their particular skills. They were able to bring to the task their understanding of the information resources available to facilitate checking, and a sophisticated ability to check databases and correct errors. At ease with the technology and quick to learn the functionality of new software, they paid attention to detail, and were able to liaise efficiently with academics, administrators and publishers. They could communicate effectively both up and down the chain of command, and showed at all times an underlying awareness that important deadlines had to be met.

For the Library team, outcomes of their involvement in the project were uniformly positive. In general, as a result of the exercise, they have found themselves recognised as having some knowledge in the field of bibliometrics, an expertise which is respected and valued by their university colleagues. Relationships established in the course of the task have lasted and developed. Having worked closely and successfully with colleagues in Research and Enterprise, they found themselves invited to participate, once the submission was completed, in discussions on whether the university should put itself forward as a REF Bibliometrics Pilot institution. In the end, the Library was centrally involved in the university's decision to do so, and was joint lead with Research and Enterprise on the university's participation in the REF Bibliometrics Pilot. Engagement with other university players at this level has been status-enhancing for the Library, which can now see itself as well integrated into the institution's research strategy. The Library was pleased, too, to have been instrumental in obtaining Glasgow University Senate approval for an institutional publications policy which requires staff to deposit the bibliographic details and full text of all peer-reviewed journal articles and conference proceedings in the university's repository, Enlighten.[6]

The institutional repository: Enlighten

The contribution made to Glasgow University's RAE submission by the Enlighten repository itself should be noted, and has been well documented by its managers, Morag Greig and William Nixon.[7] While the university did not have a central publications database in place at the time of the 2008 submission, the Library was charged with developing one after the RAE return was received. Discussions took place over whether the repository should form the basis of such a database, or whether separate software should be used to collect bibliographic details in a new one, and push data out to Enlighten, along with full text if possible. In the end, it was decided that it would be best to establish Enlighten as the only publications database, thus ensuring that academics would not be confused about the need to record their publications in two places, and allowing Enlighten to be positioned as a key university service, central to the processes of the upcoming REF. Subsequent work has secured JISC funding (via its Enrich bid) to develop the integration of Enlighten with other University systems, in particular, the Research Management System. Recognising that the repository cannot play the range of roles expected by its users and institution if it continues to exist as 'a separate and disconnected silo', the Library is currently using the funding to enhance the usability of

Enlighten for depositors by linking it to the university's research system via a single sign-on login.[8]

The role of liaison

Glasgow's experience illustrates interestingly a range of staffing grades engaged in the RAE exercise. John MacColl, in his companion report to the OCLC study, points out that libraries 'must ensure that they have a voice in the planning of institutional responses to assessment and avoid the requirement to play a merely reactive or largely clerical role'.[9] It would be true to say that while the RA2 team at the 'coal face' of the exercise contributed essential skills – checking, verification, keying, the amassing of both bibliographic details and hard copy – these might be considered inappropriate for the more senior grades at which liaison/subject librarians are normally employed. The Liaison Librarian contemplating deployment in this area would be more likely to be called upon to contribute supervisory skills, overseeing the more junior grades undertaking these tasks, and liaising with academic staff to resolve queries and difficulties. At Glasgow University, Susan Ashworth's engagement as Assistant Director with senior colleagues in the RAE, REF and Bibliometrics Working Parties was important in allowing the Library to contribute at the all-important strategic level at which university policies might be influenced and the Library's voice heard.

In general, staff of all grades at the University of Glasgow Library moved happily into this field of new challenges. New things had, of course, to be learned. While the subject librarians already had a broad understanding of bibliometrics (citation rates, Hirsch Index, impact factors, and so on), involvement in the REF Pilot required a rather more in-depth knowledge, and the small team engaged in this exercise discovered these finer details in the course of their participation – a steep, but interesting and ultimately satisfying learning curve which left them even better equipped to understand possible future developments in this area.

Though no downsides could really be identified to the University of Glasgow Library's experience of participation in the RAE, it would be important to stress that the institution's priorities have to be under constant review. Since the RAE/REF are strategically important for the university, the Library must clearly ensure that its own strategic planning and objective setting are in line with those of the university. This might result in other Library activities having to be curtailed or dropped, especially where resources are tight, in order to allow continued engagement in this new area of research support. Care would have to be taken to ensure that staff were kept informed as this process of prioritisation played out, and that they understood the need for any changes.

Lessons learned for similar projects

The importance of liaison has been at the heart of Susan's experience with the RAE. The need for the Library and its staff to connect with the university's academics was paramount to the whole operation, and, though this may have been effortful at times, the rewards were rich. The Library learned in significant ways about its research constituencies, with their subject-specific learning, teaching and publishing activities. The Library was able to connect importantly, too, with the institution's busy administrative echelons, and enjoyed opportunities for showcasing a range of bibliographic, technical and other library skills. Liaison within the Library's RAE team itself was also important, and there was undoubtedly a sense that the group which had worked so closely together for many months on such a pressurised task had 'suffered together' and bonded well – a good basis for any future working relationships.

As a project, it also foregrounded the need for strong organisational skills and a clear-sighted managerial approach which could rationalise timetables and prioritise requirements. This was a venture which could only be delivered by a good manager, one capable of setting goals, analysing tasks and pulling staff together as a group to achieve them. It demanded a range of strengths, including people-skills as well as technical and intellectual expertise. In Susan's experience, too, it was a project which required the careful synchronisation of university, RAE and Library processes, and ensured that the Library's staff learned to think usefully outside their comfortable 'library box'.

Asked for advice for anyone considering managing a Library REF team in the future, Susan said:

- Ensure that you have strong relationships with people both in relevant central university departments and with your academic community.
- Prioritise the work and create resources to support it. That might mean reprioritising of other activities.
- Establish clear processes and guidelines for the collection and administration of REF data. Ensure that these processes are supported by the institution's senior management.

Notes

1. Key Perspectives Ltd, *A Comparative Review of Research Assessment Regimes in Five Countries and the Role of Libraries in the Research Assessment Process*. Report commissioned by

OCLC Research (2009): 34. Available at: *http://www.oclc.org/research/publications/library/2009/2009-09.pdf.*

2. Ann-Marie James has written about her experiences at the University of Birmingham. Ann-Marie James, 'Dotting the DOIs and crossing the ESSNs: librarians' support for the RAE 2008', *Serials,* 21(3) (2008): 174–7. Available at: *http://dx.doi.org/10.1629/21174.* Susan Ashworth has written about Glasgow University Library's contribution. Susan Ashworth, 'Research support at the University of Glasgow Library', *SCONUL Focus,* 45 (2009): 50–1. Available at: *http://www.sconul.ac.uk/publications/newsletter/45/15.pdf.*

3. Email interview with author, February 2010.

4. Susan Ashworth, 'Research support at the University of Glasgow Library', *SCONUL Focus,* 45 (2009): 51. Available at: *http://www.sconul.ac.uk/publications/newsletter/45/15.pdf.*

5. Not everyone submitted four publications. Those with special circumstances (e.g. Early Career Researchers and those with periods of absence) could submit a reduced number.

6. University of Glasgow Publications Policy, available at: *http://www.lib.gla.ac.uk/enlighten/publicationspolicy/;* University of Glasgow Institutional Repository, Enlighten, available at: *http://www.lib.gla.ac.uk/enlighten/.*

7. Morag Greig and William Nixon, 'On the Road to Enlightenment: establishing an institutional repository service for the University of Glasgow', *OCLC Systems & Services: International Digital Library Perspectives,* 23(3) (2007): 297–309. Available at: *http://dx.doi.org/10.1108/10650750710776431.* Morag Greig, 'Achieving an "enlightened" publications policy at the University of Glasgow', *Serials* 22(1) (2009): 7–11. Available at: *http:/dx.doi.org/10/1629/227.*

8. JISC Enrich – Enhancement Strand. *Overview of University of Glasgow's Enlighten Project.* Available at: *http://www.jisc.ac.uk/whatwedo/programmes/inf11/sue2/enrich.*

9. John MacColl, *Research Assessment and the Role of the Library.* Report produced by OCLC Research (2010). Available at: *http://www.oclc.org/research/publications/library/2010/2010-01.pdf.*

Liaison and virtual worlds

Abstract: Reference and Distance Services Librarian at George Fox University's Portland Center, Oregon, USA, Robin Ashford, has been a keen early adopter of Second Life, quick to see its relevance and potential for the teaching of her distance students. Within her university's School of Education, she has had the rewarding experience of liaising with Faculty to teach and support a number of courses, mostly at graduate level. She has enjoyed developing her 'real world' librarian role within the virtual realm, providing information about resources in the many fun new ways which Second Life offers, as well as being present to help apprehensive new visitors to the world, uncertain about how to orientate themselves in this strange new environment. She also describes her experience as Consumer Health Librarian on the National Library of Medicine's Karuna Island Project, where she was able to liaise with consumer health professionals and assist with the Project's objective of compiling and developing a collection of high quality resources on AIDS/HIV.

Key words: academic liaison, case study, collaboration, distance learning, embedded librarian, faculty liaison, information literacy, Karuna Island Project, librarians, librarianship, Second Life, virtual worlds.

Virtual worlds

Robin Ashford turned enthusiastically in the new direction of Second Life in 2006, when she realised that educational institutions were seizing teaching opportunities there, and that if faculty at her own university followed suit they would be likely to need help with information resources. In 2008, when approached by a professor teaching the Educational Foundations and Leadership graduate programme at George Fox University (GFU) to assist on the course as an embedded librarian, she 'jumped in', already convinced that it was important for her to become conversant with this new technology now so central to her constituents' needs. As a 'late career librarian with an entrepreneurial background', she had always followed emergent technologies closely, and quickly saw the potential for the use of virtual worlds in her own post as Reference and Distance Services Librarian at the Portland Center of GFU.[1]

Robin found herself in summer 2008 fully integrated into EDFL 675, a graduate, one-credit hour, optional course entitled 'Faith Learning Seminar: Faith and Religious Practice Online'. The professor explained that he needed help with information resources for his students, a small group of seven, as well as general assistance with teaching basic Second Life skills. In important initial liaison conversations, he and Robin agreed on the seminar's objectives, which were:

- to learn how to survive as a resident in Second Life;
- to become familiar with basic resources for possible educational use in Second Life;
- to experience and document community life in Second Life.

Students would learn first how to create and customise their avatars, form identities, move easily (walk, transport, fly, use vehicles), communicate (instant messaging, chat, note cards, voice and offline conversations), obtain items and manage inventories, and finally search, find people, places, items, groups and information content. They would then learn how to retrieve, store and present information in Second Life, and about processes for designing and delivering instruction. This would be followed by guidance on how to use communication and social networking tools – seminars, images, models, animations and texts for information transfer. Finally, they would learn how to participate in the Second Life Community, perform group activities, learn the group culture and interact with group members. In practice, it proved impossible to meet all these objectives within the confines of a one-credit hour course, and a certain amount of rethinking was done as the course proceeded to take account of this limitation, but the exercise was useful nevertheless in allowing Robin and the professor to outline the ground they would ideally like to cover.

The synchronous parts of the course took place fully in Second Life, except for the first class, which was a face-to-face starter meeting, and a course wiki was used for the asynchronous parts. Progression into Second Life seemed natural for this course, as the professor in charge taught almost solely online for the School of Education, students coming from all over the country as well as from abroad.

A notable feature of Robin's involvement in this course was her close professional relationship with the Faculty responsible for teaching it:

> Having a close and open relationship with this faculty member was critical to the success of this project. There were no tensions/problems in this area. We regularly met on the university's Second Life skydeck to discuss how the class was going. This was new for both of us

[and] there was a lot to learn about working with students in this virtual world environment. We would discuss the feedback we were receiving from students while inworld and from their journal postings on the course wiki. At times we made changes based on the feedback to make it easier for students to accomplish their tasks.[2]

Teaching a course in Second Life: the librarian's role

Robin explains that she did not really do any formal classroom-style library teaching for this course, but created information resources and made them available, both in Second Life and on the course wiki, for the students to learn more or less on their own during times which were convenient for them. Robin also provided one-on-one live reference help when requested. Students were shown how they could contact her by having their avatar touch an object in the Second Life library building. If they were in Second Life working on their assignments and ran into problems, clicking the object immediately sent Robin a message that a student was in her office and needing assistance. If she was inside Second Life, she would receive the message instantly and could teleport from wherever she was and be on the skydeck to meet with the student within seconds. If she was busy attending an event at another university inside Second Life, she would send an instant message to notify the student of when she would be finished. If she was not in Second Life at the time the student's avatar touched the object, she would receive email notification that someone was requesting assistance. At that point she could decide whether to login to Second Life to join the student, or, if she was busy, she could reply to the email and let the student know they would need to wait or schedule for another time.

Help was, she felt, required in two main areas, namely subject-related materials required to supplement course content, and Second Life-related materials required to help students and staff orientate themselves in the virtual world. She created an office for herself on the university's skydeck, and populated it with interestingly presented help materials.[3] There were, for instance, scripted computers which connected to the George Fox Library and university homepages, and other course-specific scripted objects which could be used to assist with assignments in Second Life, all created to meet student and faculty needs. The EDFL 675 course wiki linked to round objects in Robin's skydeck office, which, when clicked, gave access to useful applications. It was possible, for instance, to order books from the online catalogue by clicking one of the objects and opening an inworld browser. Another object led to a preset search on the topic of virtual worlds in the library's consortium catalogue for students interested in learning more on this topic. Robin also supplied an intriguing green vending machine from which students were encouraged to obtain a Sloog HUD (Heads up Display), a tagging tool which allows places and avatars to be identified in Second Life. At the unique tag for EDFL 675, for example, she was able to create a set of resources required by students enrolled there – an inworld subject guide, for instance, and a complete list of the Second Life places they needed to visit for their course. Producing subject guides is, Robin feels, a particularly useful role for the Second Life librarian, providing as it does much-needed inworld support for nervous first-time visitors to the virtual realm.

Robin and the professor were both present in Second Life for each teaching session. He and she would be ready on the skydeck 15 minutes before the class start time, and as students arrived would chat informally until everyone was present – conversations would be either voice or text chat. Once the group had all appeared, they would generally teleport to another location reserved by the professor, where he would facilitate a discussion around the students' weekly assignment. (They were required to have spent one hour during the week in Second Life, visiting places, interviewing people and so on, and to have posted a journal entry about their activity on the course wiki.) After the live class time, Robin and the professor often offered the option of going back to the skydeck for more informal chat, or sometimes visiting another area in Second Life just for fun. Robin herself was frequently able to offer one-to-one help to students who were struggling with particular areas, and most took advantage of these offers, arranging times to meet with her to go over specific problems.

An important part of her role, Robin felt, was to make people comfortable with the virtual environment, and with this in mind she might take them, for example, on a shopping trip to learn some basic online skills. Accompanying them, for instance, to a freebie Second Life store, she might help them buy furniture, toys, clothes, and so on, and watch them relax and develop their inworld confidence. She might also help them upload first or Second Life snapshots of themselves to the course photoboard, thus mastering another basic skill.

Her enthusiasm for the Second Life medium was perhaps one of the main things she was able to contribute to the course. She is keen to promote the many things she feels this virtual world can offer – it allows people to connect with others from around the globe, creates a strong feeling of presence, a face-to-face experience closer to real life than other online technologies, and makes possible real-time collaboration between individuals in an environment with a strong 3-D component. It also gives people the opportunity to dream and create in an immersive, interactive learning space.

Between classes, Robin and the professor would regularly meet up on the skydeck to discuss student progress. At one point they agreed that their expectations were too high and had to be adjusted to allow students more time to master basic Second Life skills. Some really were struggling with the technology, and the orientation offered by Linden Lab in 2008 was not adequate for all. Although some students learned easily, others did not – the average age of the class was around 37, which may have been a factor. Some were attempting to access Second Life on computers which met only the minimum specifications for using it, and there were also at times issues with broadband connectivity. It was often difficult for students to find enough time simply to be in Second Life and immerse themselves in the demands of the environment. Second Life, both Robin and the professor realised, is not for everyone, and acclimatising to it frequently subjects students to a steep learning curve. Watching students tackle the tasks set for them, Robin had a sense of learning *with* the professor about how to teach in this virtual world, and that for both it was an interesting voyage of discovery.

At all points in this new venture, Robin felt her opinion was valued and that she was making a genuine contribution to the success of the course. Pleasingly, too, an additional benefit which arose from the collaboration was that it introduced them to another School of Education professor at Pacific University in Oregon, who was also interested in virtual worlds for educators. Together they wrote up, published and presented accounts of their experiences in this area at three separate, peer-reviewed educational venues.[4]

Teaching the teachers in Second Life

Following the success of her involvement with EDFL 675, Robin was delighted to be invited by the same professor to teach for a further two semesters as an adjunct instructor on the graduate course 'Introduction to Second Life for Educators' (EDFL 625).[5] The purpose of the course, conducted fully within Second Life, was to acquaint participants with the virtual world, and to discover the functions, processes and relationships which exist within it, as well as the potential of virtual worlds generally for educators and education. Participants would learn how to survive as residents in Second Life, become familiar with its educational resources, and experience community life within the Second Life environment.

Robin had sole responsibility for this course, and found herself now teaching not only five graduate students, but also six members of the School of Education staff, including the Dean – a slightly daunting prospect! It was, however, a situation which resulted in useful long-term liaison contacts, as she built up strong relationships with all faculty members, which she has continued to draw on post-course. Although she is not the official liaison librarian for the Education Department, she is regularly called on for various purposes by these faculty members as a consequence of the relationships which were forged during this time.

As with EDFL 675, the course started with an inworld 'meet and greet' session, reinforcing the basic skills for orientation, showing the importance of avatar customisation, and helping participants to establish their identity and reach a reasonable level of comfort in the new environment.[6] A visit to the Second Life Abyss Museum of Ocean Science gave an early introduction to interactivity and immersion, and a tour of ISTE (the International Society for Technology in Education) helped encourage participants to learn the value of community and the benefit of joining groups. Students were then shown a stimulating range of examples of how educators were using immersive builds in Second Life. Ohio State University's Virtual Testis Tour by Dr Douglas R. Danforth, Associate Professor, Obstetrics and Gynecology, was showcased as an instance of the use made of the medium in the training of OSU medical students, while Sheila Webber's Info Lit iSchool island was highlighted and toured as a virtual space where information science and management students receive essential aspects of their training. This space is also where regular professional development opportunities take place for librarians/educators from around the globe, often around the topic of information/digital literacy.

Virtual worlds teaching: pros and cons

Inevitably, an important aspect of this course was its attention to the theory of virtual worlds, and Robin even-handedly allowed her students to explore the debate about whether or not they add value to the educational canon.[7] Second Life triggers a lot of attention, is immersive, absorbing, inviting to explore. The environment creates enthusiasm, stimulates participation and collaboration, and must be engaged with fully if its potential is to be realised – it is as important to 'learn to live' in Second Life as it is in real life. On the other hand, for some students there is so much freedom in Second Life that it is hard to control and maintain attention. It offers so many distractions that it prevents them focusing on learning tasks. For some, the problem is that, compared with gaming, Second Life is not playful enough, offers no challenge and is not intriguing.

For those who contend that Second Life is an efficient educational tool, it could be said that learning to master the client is a meaningful activity in itself, that avatar customisation is a key to immersion and provides the student with new experiences and a sense of achievement. The more energy invested in mastering the client, the more it will become an extension to thinking and social networking skills. If, on the other hand, the user finds that it takes too long to master Second Life as a tool, this can then become an obstacle to involvement in intense and meaningful learning experiences. The complexity of the client is indeed perceived as a barrier at some level for most students and teachers. Again, too, traditional learning designs often do not seem to fit in Second Life, as the immersive environment is very different from most traditional course settings.

While Second Life does provide opportunities for simulating and social positioning, allowing users to address different learning styles and giving them unique opportunities to create, visualise and communicate themselves to the world, it would have to be conceded, however, that the learning experience it offers is often broad rather than deep, mostly just scratching the surface of real knowledge and understanding. It is not on the whole a provocative or rich learning environment, and large group learning activities attempted there can easily degenerate into a circus.

The Karuna Island Project

Robin's experience of teaching in virtual worlds has also extended into the area of medical science, where she was able to develop her liaison skills by working not only with academics but also with the public, other consumer and health professionals, and institutions such as AIDs.org, the

National Library of Medicine and other government agencies. From May 2009 to May 2010 she held the contract position of Consumer Health Librarian on the Karuna Island Project, a venture funded by the National Library of Medicine with support from the Alliance Library System. The objectives of the Karuna Project were to develop and compile a collection of high quality resources on AIDS/HIV, to make these easily accessible and ensure that people were aware of them, to train patients and their families in how to search for information on all aspects of the disease, and to collaborate with other AIDS/HIV health information agencies to provide a high standard of material. Inspired by and committed to this worthwhile project, Robin proceeded to create the Karuna Resource Center, where she enjoyed establishing a relaxed, comfortable Second Life environment in which enquirers could meet to share experience, give presentations, collaborate and converse.[8] Information, mostly derived from government agencies, was attractively and accessibly stored in a variety of clickable displays around the room. When touched, these would either release an information notecard or open up an inworld web-browser which could also be opened in an external browser for later reference. PowerPoint viewers enabled the showing of presentations on, for example, how to search Medline Plus for information on AIDS/HIV, while a large round ball in the centre of the room could be clicked for access to the substantial and comprehensive WHO/UNAIDS report. Users reported that they enjoyed this quirky, slightly challenging approach to information retrieval, and appreciated the laidback anonymity of the immersive environment.

Robin found her time with the Karuna Island Project 'a truly remarkable experience', which extended her understanding of virtual worlds and convinced her more than ever that these can have valuable educational and therapeutic roles to play.[9] She has blogged and taught enthusiastically about *How Doctors, Nurses, Allied Health Professionals and Patients Use Second Life*, and was able to bring back to her academic post an even fuller grasp of the contribution Second Life can make in this area.[10]

Robin has taught most recently (Autumn 2010) on her university's MLDR 550 Communications in Ministry course, which was slightly different from others in which she has been involved in that it was taught by two adjuncts, one of whom was a well-known author. She again collaborated closely with the hybrid learning director and one of the adjuncts to ensure that her teaching fulfilled the needs of the course. This careful liaison with faculty regarding the content of her teaching was again, she found, critical to the success of her role on the course.[11]

Other virtual worlds roles for librarians?

Robin's experience of virtual worlds has been both extensive and varied, and she is herself proof perfect of the value of the information skills support role which librarians can play within these environments. Are there any other roles she sees librarians fulfilling there in the future? There are, she confirms, a few 'very techie librarians who have created amazing builds in Second Life', and points to the Tintern Abbey build undertaken by reference librarian and Assistant Professor Denise Cote at College of DuPage, Glen Ellyn, Illinois.[12] The advanced skills required for projects at this level can be obtained by taking the relevant classes in Second Life, but in Robin's experience most of the advanced work of this kind she has seen by librarians has been done by those who already had programming skills when they first

entered. Most academic librarians she has encountered in
Second Life

> are there to offer support via a Second Life library or
> sometimes in very creative spaces where they hold
> events for their universities and provide access to
> information resources and are there to assist as the
> needs arise as I've done on our university skydeck.[13]

Refreshed within this new twenty-first-century virtual
context, the traditional liaison role of support and assistance
is revalidated and confirmed as crucial to the learning
experience.

  Is this a new direction for liaison librarians which Robin
sees as developing in the future? It is possibly too early to
say. Things change fast in virtual worlds, and it may be that
this is an idea which has come and gone for some academic
librarians. The dominance of Second Life in the virtual arena
has waned significantly since around 2009, and more so
since Linden Lab announced the end of educational discounts
in 2010 – interestingly, the George Fox skydeck was deleted
from Second Life in June 2011. Even so, Robin is convinced
that there is still continual and important growth taking
place in the virtual world arena. She quotes the Kzero
website's assertion that 'the virtual worlds sector now has
1.4 billion cumulative registered accounts', and their recent
Q2 2011 data which shows the largest quarterly increase in
take-up in this area since they began tracking in 2008.[14] She
notes the 615 million in the 10–15-year-old age group who
are registered users of virtual worlds, and who will be
entering Higher Education in the next five to ten years. Used
to gaming and social media of all kinds, and to interacting
with engaging systems throughout the day, these young
people will reach university with no expectation of being

taught there by the traditional 'sage on a stage' lecture approach. Although she cannot predict precisely how things will develop, she is sure that this upcoming generation, with its problem-solving and critical thinking skills honed through continual engagement with the gaming and social media environments, will be well equipped for involvement in virtual worlds, and will be excited by the evolution of augmented reality, the 3-D web and immersive systems generally.

Her own engagement with virtual worlds has been an important experiment very much worth undertaking, and she has been inspired by the experience. Librarians of all kinds, she believes, can benefit tremendously from the professional development opportunities this area affords. 'The ability to connect and collaborate on a global level continues to be of great value to me. I have not yet found another technology that comes close to VWs in this area.'[15] She is also acutely aware that her involvement, and the development of her skills, have been crucial to the teaching and learning needs of her university's staff and students. She feels obliged

> to go where those at my institution are teaching and learning. According to my library's mission statement we are, 'to support the instructional programs and research activities of our institutions by providing access to information in a variety of formats, and to provide instruction in the use of traditional and new information and technologies.' What I have done as a librarian in Second Life lines up with my library's mission statement.[16]

She knows, too, that in this age of digital revolution librarians must adapt or die.

At a time when the relevance of librarians is being scrutinized, I can't imagine saying 'no' to a professor who asks if a librarian can assist with the information needs of a course being taught in a virtual world, inside a course management system such as Moodle or Blackboard, or on a social networking site such as Facebook or Twitter. My answer has always been 'Yes, I'm glad to help.' If I'm asked to use a technology I'm not familiar with to assist with a class, I know now more than ever that I can learn it. (Experience in virtual worlds can do that to a person).[17]

Liaison librarians who, like Robin, cross either enthusiastically or with trepidation into the arena of virtual worlds, will prove themselves alert to change, adaptable and quick to learn. The students and Faculty who receive their help there will surely be grateful for it.

Lessons learned for similar projects

Robin's enthusiasm for her virtual worlds projects is inspiring. She is excited to be involved in this medium, and thrives on the pleasure of teaching herself how to operate in virtual worlds and get the most out of them. The vigour with which she approaches the learning challenge is refreshing, and it is to a large extent her openness and honesty about her sometimes apprehensive self-taught status which make her such a good teacher of others. She reassures the faltering novice to the virtual world and normalises the uncertainty of the experience. We share her delight in learning new things and extending her librarian's horizons.

She is keen to emphasise the value of community in virtual worlds, seeing them perhaps as useful microcosms of the real world, in which it is important to make connections with others, share experience and develop understanding through interaction. For her, virtual worlds offer liaison opportunities at the most essential level. She urges the newcomer to attend inworld events, to draw on what other people have learned and made available to them, and not to be concerned about initial slow progress. She is an empathetic teacher, keen to encourage involvement but realistic about possible difficulty. Like E.M. Forster in *Howards End*, her motto is 'Only connect.'

Robin's advice for liaison librarians setting out on a virtual world project:

- Gain a good understanding of the Second Life culture and a strong level of expertise in at least the basics of Second Life before embarking on any kind of project. Having a good handle on basic Second Life skills such as navigating, communicating, camera controls, maps, group notifications, etc. is critical before starting. Before taking on any kind of project or even a major role in assisting a class as I did as a liaison librarian, it's important to be comfortable in the VW yourself. From my experience, the best way to do this is to enter Second Life and attend events. I strongly recommend becoming involved in librarian and other educator groups already working/playing/learning in the VW. Educator groups such as ISTE (International Society for Technology in Education) and Community Virtual Library (CVL) groups and others hold many events and have people willing to help those new to Second Life.

- When embarking on a work-related VW project, be realistic about the amount of time needed. Once a person has the basics of Second Life, and has been attending events put on by others in the educational community, it becomes easier to estimate how long it might take to put a project together. Consulting with others inworld who have done similar projects is also helpful.

- Expect to be challenged. If you're embarking on a VW project, or even just entering a VW for the first time, view it as a learning/stretching professional development opportunity for yourself.

Notes

1. Robin Ashford, Blogger profile. Available at: *http://www.blogger.com/profile/04867035352518158417*.
2. Email interview with author, July 2011.
3. See Robin's PowerPoint presentation, *An Academic Librarian in Second Life*, available at: *http://www.slideshare.net/RobinAshford/academic-librarian-in-second-life-presentation*, and slides of EDFL 675 in Second Life available at: *http://www.flickr.com/photos/25095603@N07/sets/72157606936878733/*.
4. R. Ashford, S. Headley, and A. Zijdemans-Boudreau, 'Do educators need a Second Life? Exploring possibilities for technology-based distance learning in higher education', in I. Gibson et al. (eds), *Proceedings of Society for Information Technology and Teacher Education International Conference* (Chesapeake, VA: AACE, 2009): 1617–22. Available at: *http://www.editlib.org/p/30846*. R. Ashford, S. Headley, and A. Zijdemans-Boudreau, 'Immersive virtual worlds in educational practice: introducing educators to Second Life', in T. Bastaiens et al. (eds), *Proceedings of World Conference on E-Learning in Corporate, Government, Healthcare, and Higher Education* (Chesapeake, VA: AACE, 2009): 2076–81. Available at: *http://www.editlib.org/p/32770*. R. Ashford, S. Headley, and A. Zijdemans-Boudreau, 'Faculty preparation for teaching and learning in Second Life', in T. Bastiaens et al. (eds), *Proceedings of World Conference on E-Learning in Corporate, Government, Healthcare, and Higher Education* (Chesapeake, VA: AACE, 2009): 2366–8. Available at: *http://www.editlib.org/p/32814*.

5. George Fox University, Course EDFL 625. Available at: *http://introto2ndlifeforeducators.pbworks.com/w/page/20127992/FrontPage*.
6. For slides of EDFL 625 in Second Life, see: *http://www.flickr.com/photos/25095603@N07/sets/72157614072305900/*.
7. See Robin's PowerPoint presentation, *Informal Adult Learning in Second Life*. Available at: *http://www.slideshare.net/RobinAshford/informal-adult-learning-in-second-life*.
8. See Robin's PowerPoint presentation, *A Consumer Health Librarian's National Library of Medicine Funded Project in Second Life*. Available at: *http://www.slideshare.net/RobinAshford/consumer-health-librarianinsecondlifefinal*.
9. Email interview with author, July 2011.
10. See Robin's Posterous Blog. Available at: *http://robinashford.posterous.com/tag/karunaresourcecenter*, as well as her Librarian By Design Blog, *http://librarianbydesign.blogspot.com/search/label/karuna*. Also her PowerPoint presentation, *How Doctors, Nurses, Allied Health Professionals and Patients Use Second Life*. Available at: *http://www.slideshare.net/RobinAshford/how-doctors-nurses-allied-health-professionals-and-patients*.
11. For slides of MLDR 550 in Second Life, see: *http://www.flickr.com/photos/25095603@N07/sets/72157625447837867/*.
12. College of DuPage Newsroom, 'College uses Second Life to educate students', 16 November 2009. Available at: *http://triblocal.com/glen-ellyn/community/stories/2009/11/college-uses-second-life-to-educate-students/*.
13. Email interview with author, July 2011.
14. Kzero website. Available at: *http://www.kzero.co.uk/blog/?p=4625*.
15. Email interview with author, August 2011.
16. Email interview with author, August 2011.
17. Email interview with author, August 2011.

4

Liaison and digital scholarship

Abstract: This chapter offers three case studies of librarians involved in collaborative digitisation projects. Two former liaison librarians at the University of Sydney Library manage the Australian Poetry Resource Library (APRIL), which makes available on the internet a wide range of original material for Australian poets. Ross Coleman describes the project's set-up and procedures. At the University of Glasgow Library, former subject librarian Dr Stephen Rawles became involved in the Glasgow Emblem Digitisation Project, producing an impressive full-text database of emblem-book material from his library's Stirling Maxwell Collection. At California Digital Library, Lisa Schiff describes the origins of the Mark Twain Papers Project emanating from the University of Berkeley's Bancroft Library. The chapter suggests that liaison librarians of the future might enter the profession with new qualifications in Digital Humanities scholarship.

Key words: academic liaison, APRIL Project, California Digital Library, copyright, digitisation, electronic publishing, e-scholarship, faculty liaison, Glasgow Emblem Digitisation Project, Mark Twain Papers and Project, scholarly communication, Sydney Digital Library, University of Glasgow Library, University of Sydney Library.

'Libraries used to be scholar-centred and are now information-centred, and they need to be moving back to be scholar-centred and working out what users really want, as well as promoting what they do,' says Christine Madsen, first Balliol-Bodley scholar at the University of Oxford, interviewed in *Floreat Domus, Balliol College News*.[1] Increasing numbers of librarians are recognising the truth of this observation, and are devoting their energies to providing support in the areas where their scholars really want it. As researchers become more and more dependent on electronic resources, librarians are moving with growing enthusiasm in the new direction of e-scholarship and developing the new support skills and services demanded by their digitally alert academic community. The value of libraries' digital repositories to scholarly exercises such as the UK REF has been referred to in Chapter 2 and extensively documented elsewhere, but the current chapter will highlight some examples of librarians making even more ambitious and carefully tailored digital provision for their clientele. Librarians' involvement in digitisation projects of various kinds is becoming both increasingly sophisticated and driven by user need.

The Australian Poetry Library, University of Sydney

At the University of Sydney, librarians have been quick to focus their services on what their scholars really want. Managed by two former Faculty Liaison Librarians, the Australian Poetry Resources Internet Library (now renamed the Australian Poetry Library, but earlier known by its acronym, APRIL) satisfies genuine scholarly need by making available on the internet a wide range of original literary material from Australian poets, providing access to impressive numbers of primary texts, reviews, memoirs, diaries, interviews, audio and visual materials.[2] Working collaboratively with writers, academic scholars and copyright experts, these librarians have realised their vision of creating a database of immense value to the scholarly community.

The project began in 2004 as a prototype internet site entitled 'Australian Literature Resources' designed and built by the poet John Tranter and sponsored by Australian Literary Management. In 2006, the site featured material relating to around 70 poets, and attracted a substantial grant from the Australian Research Council to facilitate its further development. A project team was then put in place, headed by Professor Elizabeth Webber at the University of Sydney's English Department, and involving both Dr Creagh Cole and Ross Coleman of the University of Sydney Library, along with the Copyright Agency Limited (CAL) as a linkage partner, and John Tranter in a consulting role. By February 2010, over 42,000 poems had been processed and added to the site, and the project is now well on its way to delivering free viewing of all APRIL material in HTML or PDF format. A transactionally based e-commerce system currently administered by the Copyright Agency Limited allows fees to be paid to authors and other copyright holders for any material downloaded or printed.

APRIL, as Ross Coleman confirms, is the culmination of many earlier University of Sydney Library projects where skills, facilities and collaborations were developed.[3] His 2008 article gives a comprehensive and inspiring overview of how librarians at Sydney have developed a framework of eScholarship activities incorporating digital collections, open access repositories, eResearch data services and a scholarly publication platform.[4] Their Sydney Electronic Text and Image Service (SETIS) was established in the mid-1990s, initially with the aim of networking commercial full-text databases such as the *Thesaurus Linguae Graecae* and

Patrologia Latina, but quickly evolving into a platform for the creation of text and image-based digital collections. The first major SETIS project was the production of full-text primary and secondary texts for the Australian Research Council-funded AUSTLIT database.[5] More than 300 works of Australian fiction and poetry ranging from the early nineteenth century to the 1930s were digitised (XML, TEI tagged), along with a large number of critical materials relating to Australian authors and their works. This impressive operation allowed Sydney to demonstrate its expertise in the role of textual conversion to eHumanities standards, and to establish itself as the leader in the field of full-text management, thus opening the way for creating a publishing operation to satisfy the demand for print versions.

In 2003, the university re-registered the previously abandoned imprint of Sydney University Press under Library management, with the new aim of addressing the challenges of scholarly publication in the internet environment. SUP now functions as a successful commercial publisher, publishing in short runs and on a print on demand basis new titles approved by an editorial board, as well as a growing reprint list. The SUP archives are stored in the Sydney eScholarship Repository, another arm of the integrated eScholarship network. This DSpace installation provides a secure open access repository service and allows the SUP publishing venture to be complemented by open access publishing activities. Sydney digital theses, SETIS digital collections, the eScholarship repository and other advisory and hosting services all function under the umbrella of the Sydney Digital Library and operate in partnership with Sydney University Publishing. The synergy produced by these integrated activities results in the creation and availability of high-quality scholarly materials genuinely desired by the academic community. Scholars articulate their demands, and Sydney eScholarship produces.

The involvement of two former Faculty Liaison Librarians in the APRIL project is interesting evidence of spheres of activity changing to meet perceived new needs. Staff have been moved from traditional roles to new ones in response to evolving demands. Three library staff members work directly on the project and two others are associated with it. An HEO (Higher Education Officer) at Level 6 (base rate for professional librarian) is employed half-time as Digital Production Coordinator; an HEO 7 Development Programmer works 1–2 days per week; and the HEO 8 SETIS Coordinator oversees the overall architecture of the project and undertakes the actual coding of the files, 1–2 days per week. The Digital Production Coordinator and SETIS Coordinator are former Faculty Liaison Librarians. Associated with the project are the HEO 9 Business Manager of Sydney University Press, who advises on scoping the publishing of customized anthologies, and the HEO 10 internal business owner of the project, who is also on the project steering group.

The Library's contribution to the project is both technical and intellectual. The editorial selection of poets to be included in the database is made by Professor Elizabeth Webber, assisted by John Tranter, but the final say on inclusion rests with the poets themselves, who have to agree to the arrangements for their remuneration. Library staff have marginal input to this stage of the process, but are part of the review process, and contribute to discussions relating to conceptual design, metadata, textual tagging and the visual presentation of poetical works.

The workflow starts with the physical selection of material. All editions of an individual poet's work are identified for digitisation, sometimes excluding complete or collected works, as these are often reprints. Digital conversion is then carried out by a vendor in Mumbai, India, who double-keys materials and delivers them in an XML DTD established by Sydney University Library. The received files are checked for accuracy, processed according to the general bibliographic architecture of the database, then uploaded for tagging. Works are tagged for general presentation (collections, poems, titles, stanzas, first lines, gender, year, etc., as well as for free keyword searching). Files are then tagged for presentation, and links made between poems, biographies and multimedia. Site and functional design is being implemented using XTF (eXtensible Text Framework) developed by California Digital Library. The XTF site exists in tandem with the new Australian Poetry Library site (designed for a more dynamic commercial look), and continues to function as the master digital archive.

With almost two-thirds of the poets signed up for the database still alive, copyright is obviously a major issue. Library staff are not involved in this area, which is dealt with entirely by CAL – a substantial contribution to the project, as they manage the contracts of all poets and agents involved, and resolve all related matters.

Writing applications for funding for APRIL, as with other Sydney eScholarship projects, has been a responsibility shared between the Library and academic staff. Since an academic research outcome is always required, the final submission is seen as a faculty responsibility, but with Library input – an important area for collaboration.

Moving into this new arena of digital expertise has been viewed positively by staff, and brought a sense of satisfaction – even excitement – to those involved, as reflected in the extensive writing and reporting on the venture by project staff.[6] Inevitably, though, some issues continue to present challenges. Work continues on the further refinement of the database's functionality, especially with regard to advanced and comparative searches. The processing, encoding and rendering of poems which are idiosyncratic in their word arrangement, spacing, formatting and style remain sometimes problematic, and there are potentially still some issues around disabling technologies to protect on-screen content. Audio and video functionality has still to be embedded, and there is some ironing out to be done of problems relating to custom anthologisation techniques, costing and printing on demand. Prices for the downloading and printing of material have still to be finalised, though the technicalities have been resolved and put in place by CAL. Arrangements have also still to be confirmed about how search engines or literature services will discover or link to poems at poem level, and other publishing options such as services to schools have yet to be explored. Work is never complete on a project of this magnitude, and staff look set to meet all future challenges with enthusiasm and dedication.

APRIL's success provides a striking demonstration of how the extension of the Faculty Liaison Librarian's role into the digital eScholarship area can allow a Library to add value and scholarly focus to its services. That two former Faculty Liaison Librarians should have been selected to be so heavily involved in this and similar Sydney projects is significant – testimony, maybe, to the technical and collaborative skills they may be seen to bring to the job. Within the Sydney eScholarship network of services as a whole, five staff are ex-Faculty Liaison Librarians, a situation which illustrates the perhaps inevitable transition of such staff to these roles. Some current Sydney Liaison Librarians have also expressed interest in being involved in digital creation projects, but demands and priorities of other work have meant that they have been unable to commit the time which projects such as APRIL require. The possibility of allowing them to be seconded temporarily to such areas is under consideration.

Glasgow Emblem Digitisation Project, University of Glasgow

The University of Glasgow offers another instance of a librarian who has made the leap into the digital arena. Dr Stephen Rawles came to the Glasgow Emblem Digitisation Project via a research background in scholarly bibliography (his 1976 Warwick PhD thesis was entitled *Denis Janot, Parisian printer and bookseller (fl. 1529–1544): a bibliographic study*) and his post as subject librarian and Senior Cataloguer for the Humanities Division at Glasgow University Library. His interest in Emblem literature was long-standing, usefully fuelled by the extensive, world-leading collection of emblem books in GUL's Stirling Maxwell Collection. Drawing on these rich resources in his own library, Stephen first of all worked with Professor Alison Adams of Glasgow's Department of French and Professor Alison Saunders of the University of Aberdeen to produce between 1999 and 2002 the impressive two-volume *Bibliography of French Emblem Books*, which was published by Droz and enthusiastically received by the Emblem literature community.[7]

In June 2001, his co-author and Director of the Centre of Emblem Studies Alison Adams organised a meeting in Glasgow of around 20 researchers in the field to discuss a CD-ROM digital emblem project. The workshop brought together specialists with expertise in the French, German, Dutch and Spanish emblem corpora, as well as those with knowledge of the relevant digitisation technologies, and the discussion centred on various needs. It would be necessary to develop a core set of standards for digital emblem books, to define a primary corpus of texts for digitisation, to ensure that all intellectual property issues were addressed, and to contact other scholars in the area to alert them to the potential of the new project.

In the course of an intensive but rewarding two-day programme of discussions, a number of decisions were taken:

- A core set of 100 titles would be selected from the entire European emblem corpus, based on their importance for the development of the emblem as a genre in the sixteenth and seventeenth centuries.

- Books would be digitised on a page-by-page basis. Glasgow University Library (GUL) would decide which archival format suited best, but the images would be published as JPEGs. GUL would supply most of the books for digitisation, but some gaps might need to be filled through negotiated use of volumes from other collections.

- As many full texts as possible would be published with the scanned images in order to allow full-text searching.

- With regard to image description, it was felt that the ICONCLASS classification system on balance would bring more benefits than natural language description.[8]

- Dissemination of information: information about the project would be made known to the emblem community via a Newsletter report and a mailing list.

Follow-up meetings were held in Palma in October 2001 and in Wolfenbuttel in 2003 and the project proceeded to its first phase, the production of a CD containing scanned images with a minimum of indexing. In the meantime, Rawles had produced a prototype metadata framework for digitised emblems.[9] In September 2004, however, the venture took a huge leap forward when (after an earlier unsuccessful bid) the Glasgow Centre for Emblem Studies was awarded a grant of £163,385 by the Arts and Humanities Research Council (AHRC). Under the Directorship of Professor Alison Adams, the project now turned its attention to the more ambitious and technically updated goal of 'a sophisticated website including high quality images of some 5500 pages, fully searchable text, and a full apparatus of indexes for both text and images'.[10] Two librarians held Associate and Assistant Director posts in the project respectively: David Weston, Head of Special Collections at Glasgow University Library, and Stephen Rawles, recently retired from his position as Principal Assistant Librarian, Art and Humanities. The project was managed by post doctoral research assistant Jonathan Spangler.

As Director, Alison Adams had the role of principal investigator, so she was the official grant-holder, and the AHRC money was awarded to her via the Faculty of Arts. Stephen Rawles, however, was responsible for the internal financial housekeeping and gained new skills liaising with the Finance Office to ensure that funds were husbanded and allocated without undue bureaucracy. The project was also associated with the EU-funded Study and Digitisation of Italian Emblems Project, in which Adams, Rawles and Weston are listed as Supervisor, Expert Advisor and Bibliographical Supervisor respectively, and with the later Alciato at Glasgow project, funded by the British Academy.[11]

Rawles describes the project team as 'necessarily close knit, adaptable, and got on well with itself'.[12] There was an interesting mix of technical and scholarly skills. The Computing Officers were Arts computing experts who quickly immersed themselves in the emblem environment and assimilated the project-critical data. An expert web designer enhanced the functionality of the resulting website 'beyond the dreams' of its directors, and the Project Manager, a postdoctoral student with an academic background in the history of early-modern France, also learned all he needed to know about emblems 'pdq' and ran an impressively tight project ship. Two research assistants undertook the keyboarding material, and were partially responsible for indexing using ICONCLASS, proof correction and keeping statistics. While it had been hoped initially that the encoding of modern spellings for the early-modern French could have been handled by the research assistants, this did not in the end prove possible, and was done by Adams and Rawles. The difficulty of finding someone with the necessary understanding of Latin was another hurdle to be crossed – again not something that could be handled by the research assistants. The English translation of Latin was largely out-sourced. Rawles did find himself learning some new skills, 'but nothing I would call earth-shaking', he says, since the technical support was so good. He and Adams did of necessity contribute quite significantly to the XML coding stage of the project in the difficult areas of French, Latin and Greek spellings, and found the process 'fiddly' but basically straightforward.

'It cannot be emphasised enough,' says Rawles, 'that this project worked because we did a lot of groundwork, had strong (indeed international) support from others in the emblem community (notably others in similar projects) and made it our business to cooperate with the other projects, especially to avoid reinventing the wheel!'[13] The project benefitted, as its website confirms, from initial training and ongoing help via contributions in kind from the Constantijn Huygens Institute in the Netherlands, Utrecht University, and the Memorial University of Newfoundland. It was also undertaken within the Open Emblem Initiative.[14]

Infrastructural support for the project (machines, server space, etc.) was provided by Glasgow's Humanities Advanced Technology and Information Institute (HATII), and Rawles continues to be closely associated with this group as an Honorary Research Fellow – a good example of a librarian liaising with the academic community and in due course being assimilated into it.[15] Established in 1997, HATII is internationally recognised for its interdisciplinary research in

Digital Curation, Digital Humanities, Theoretical Approaches to Information, the Philosophy of Technology, and Archives, Records and Information Management. It offers professional Masters degrees in Information Management and Preservation (ARA/SoA and CILIP accredited), Museum Studies, Computer Forensics and E-Discovery as well as a joint Honours undergraduate degree in Arts and Media Informatics and a 'dynamic interdisciplinary doctoral programme'. In content and ethos HATII seems to occupy common ground with Trinity College, Dublin's Long Room Hub and new M.Phil. in Digital Humanities and Culture, as well as with Oxford's Digital Humanities centre.[16]

Although none of the computing or technical team members on Glasgow's Emblem Project were graduates of HATII programmes, Rawles agrees that future graduates of the Institute would surely be good candidates for similar projects. Its CILIP accredited Masters degree in Information Management and Preservation would certainly be a good qualification for librarians looking to offer a specialism in digitisation skills.

Did Rawles think there might in future be more roles for subject librarians with suitable subject expertise in this kind of project? 'Not every day of the week!' is his realistic response. He is keen to emphasise that the Glasgow Emblem Digitisation venture was very *sui generis*, the result of the right books and the relevant scholarly skills coinciding in the right place at a time when the AHRC was favouring digital enterprise. This *is* a future direction worth exploring by subject/liaison librarians, but realistically only if they have the correct expertise and are in a place with the right kind of collection. 'For example, say you had a neo-Latinist subject-librarian at St Andrews who was fixated about George Buchanan, and someone gave you the dosh, and you thought there was a market, then that could be profitable . . .'[17]

Clearly his own experience with the Glasgow Emblems has been deeply satisfying and worthwhile, and offers an encouraging example of a librarian extending his traditional skills into non-traditional areas, mastering, for instance, the intricacies of XML and text-encoding. Perhaps paradoxically, too, it is an experience which exemplifies the need for both the very traditional skills of the subject librarian – Rawles is, like some of his other colleagues at Glasgow University Library, a scholar librarian *par excellence* – and the newer, technical skills now increasingly acquired by librarians to support digital literacy. Intriguingly, this is a project in which old and new library worlds meet.

Mark Twain Papers and Project, California Digital Library

Sitting interestingly alongside the Glasgow Emblem Project as a variant example of a library digitisation venture is the Mark Twain Papers and Project (MTPP) at Berkeley's Bancroft Library.[18] This digital critical edition of the writings of Mark Twain was first released to the public in October 2007, the result of several years of close collaboration between the Papers' staff at the Bancroft, the California Digital Library and the University of California Press. For that initial release, the Bancroft Library provided the content and some technical expertise, the University of California Press provided the imprint, placing the project on a par with its traditional and highly respected print offerings, and California Digital Library provided core technical skills, information architecture and design resources. As the website confirms, the first release of the Mark Twain Project Online consists of correspondence, providing access to more than 2300 complete texts, over 28,000 records of other items, and almost 100 facsimile images. The project moves beyond traditional publishing models by allowing a wider range of scholarly enquirers access to more, and more frequently updated, materials than would be available through traditional print archives, and offers advanced search facilities within the texts themselves. The digital edition also makes it possible for the edited text to be displayed alongside the editorial notes and other textual apparatus.

The Mark Twain Papers are interesting in that, as a project, it emanates from within a library, and is essentially managed by library staff. Although, as Lisa Schiff of CDL confirms, none of those involved is actually qualified as a librarian, the MTPP team operates within the Bancroft Library and its members are therefore classed in a wider sense as 'library staff'. The Papers' curator Robert Hirst is an adjunct professor at the University of Berkeley, California, his duties including occasional undergraduate teaching, and the three other most recent members of staff on the team, hired in 2005 and 2006, hold doctoral degrees in the relevant specialist areas – they have no teaching duties. Structurally this set-up, common in US libraries, might be seen to provide a useful paradigm for developing UK activities in this area. The Library absorbs and accommodates the team members with their distinctive academic and technical skills, provides the raw material for their digital editing work and, importantly, is associated with the quality digital outcome. While it does not offer an example of specifically liaison librarians moving into the digital publishing area – examples of this are surprisingly difficult to find – the MTPP project at the Bancroft does show a library as a whole embracing the concept and both accommodating and valorising the specialist staff required to move significantly forward in this direction.

The Mark Twain Papers seem to have created their own imperative. Their existence demanded a digital project and their hosting Library, recognising this, drew to itself the necessary specialist manpower. As Lisa Schiff explains, the MTPP team required people with 'advanced academic backgrounds (e.g. doctorates)' who understood the scholarly communication needs of researchers, and this team's skill sets were crucially complemented by those of a group from California Digital Library with a similar background:

> So we were all able to work together to determine what the requirements were for researchers, and then go from there to determine how to support that. MTPP technical staff were able to modify the encoded texts in order to support the citation functionality, and the CDL technical staff were able to generate the XSLT code to process and display that information appropriately. This combination of skills was also valuable for working out facet behaviour and advanced search functionality.[19]

This was not a case where existing staff had to learn new skills or adapt to new procedures. Those working on both MTPP and CDL teams had already been trained in the necessary skills either as part of their MLIS degrees or in previous employment, while others were originally programmers who had come to the library world later in their careers.

Using the skills of both teams, the texts were encoded according to the Text Encoding Initiative standard (TEI), the widely accepted set of XML guidelines and conventions for describing texts for processing by computers. Basic encoding of the letters and literary works was outsourced to a third party, who worked against a set of detailed guidelines established by MTPP staff at the Bancroft. They had to determine how to express the editorial signs and indicators in the TEI coding of the text. They also had to apply a good set of descriptive metadata to each content object, and to move these from the separate databases in which they had originally been stored into a single, rationalised and consistent one. Metadata records were generated from that database and expressed according to METS (the Metadata Encoding and Transmission Standard), a standard widely used for capturing and sharing metadata about numerous types of objects.

Interestingly, the project exists surprisingly independently of Faculty involvement. Where UK projects of this kind seem on the whole to be initiated by members of academic staff and to depend on those staff winning external funding before they can proceed to the technical, text-encoding stage, the MTPP is answerable largely to the National Endowment for the Humanities, from which most of its funding derives. Staff on the team submit a grant application to the NEH every two years, the project having an impressive track record in terms of the number of years it has received awards. The Curator, Robert Hirst, also works with Bancroft and campus-wide development staff to contact potential donors (e.g. foundations such as the Koret and private individuals), since the NEH awards scheme requires substantial matching funds, without which NEH itself gives nothing.[20] The MTPP site does not currently have a cost-recovery model, and is available without charge to anyone who wishes to use it.

The project is notable, too, for the print spin-offs it has triggered. Primarily, of course, a digital product, it has nevertheless engaged comfortably with the print world, with which it is also associated through University of California Press. In May 2011, the site advertises for sale print volumes of *The Mark Twain Papers* (scholarly editions of previously unpublished notebooks, journals, letters and manuscripts), *The Works of Mark Twain* (scholarly editions of previously published literary works) and *The Mark Twain Library* (popularly priced editions with texts, illustrations and explanatory notes, suitable for classroom use), while a print edition of *The Autobiography of Mark Twain*, Volume 1 was announced for sale in November 2010. Also available are items in the *Jumping Frogs* series, undiscovered, rediscovered and celebrated writings of Mark Twain, and Robert Hirst's own *Who Is Mark Twain?* published by Harper Studio in conjunction with the Mark Twain Project. It is interesting to see a traditional University Press being strengthened and receiving an element of future-proofing through its 'extended family' of digital scholarship projects. Print and digital media remain mutually nourishing and closely intertwined.

Lessons learned for similar projects

What advice can be offered to library teams wishing to embark on digital projects such as these successful ones at Sydney, Glasgow and Berkeley?

All involved in these case studies agree on the overriding importance of preparation – the 'pre-work' required for each of their projects has proved almost more crucial than the established 'up and running' stages. The selection of material, the preparation of data, the clarification and ordering of work flows must all be settled before the project is launched. Finance must be secured and realistic deadlines and delivery dates decided. The project's infrastructure must be robust and dependable.

A non-insular approach, too, is vital. Each practitioner interviewed has stressed the importance of getting others involved and not unnecessarily shouldering responsibility for tasks which might better be delegated or outsourced. It is important to check what others are doing, not to redo groundwork which has already been done, and to draw on other people's expertise where it is practical and affordable to do so. If working collaboratively, the individual responsibilities of partners must be clarified, while other people need to be involved also in the important stage of user testing. The project team should not be operating in a vacuum, but should be outward-looking and energised by the contributions of others. Above all, perhaps, teams should keep in mind the requirements of the end-users at whom the digital projects are aimed, and should maintain a constant dialogue with them to ensure that they are on course to deliver what is wanted.

Ross Coleman (University of Sydney Library):

- Be sure you can deliver what you promise, and cost as accurately as possible.

- Remember that actual digitisation is only a small part of the project – pre-digitisation material preparation, data-processing, file structuring, applying metadata, naming, tagging and rendering to presentation are expensive.

- Be patient – it takes time to build the skills and expertise to run such a project. While some work can be out-sourced, in-house expertise is critical.

Stephen Rawles (HATII, University of Glasgow):

- Do a lot of groundwork (e.g. our 2001 work was central to knowing what we should be doing, and what others were doing).

- If anyone else is working in the same field, contact them, cooperate and profit from joint experience – don't set up in competition. The chances are they will be glad to know someone else is looking at the same problems, with similar ends in mind. Put it another way: make sure you do not reinvent the wheel.

- Don't necessarily expect to be able to find any expertise in Latin and Greek over and above what you know you can count on locally.

Lisa Schiff (California Digital Library):

- Do an assessment of your data before starting and determine the degree of data cleansing and normalisation that is required.

- Identify the primary use cases and make sure that decisions around the design and the implementation of the site always prioritise the success of those central examples. Additionally, do user testing as early in the development as possible.

- Clarify from the outside what each partner in the collaboration will be responsible for, which areas will be shared responsibilities and establish clear timeframes with sufficient buffers for handling the unexpected.

Notes

1. Christine Madsen, interviewed by Jacqueline Smith, in 'Buried treasure', *Floreat Domus; Balliol College News*, 16 (2010): 46.
2. Australian Poetry Library, available at: *http://www.poetrylibrary.edu.au/*.
3. Email interview with author, February 2010.
4. Ross Coleman, 'Scholarly Publishing Within an eScholarship Framework – Sydney eScholarship as a Model of Integration and Sustainability', *Open Scholarship: Authority, Community and Sustainability in the Age of Web 2.0, EIPub 2008, 12th International Conference on Electronic Publishing*, Toronto, Canada, June 2008. Available at: *http://hdl.handle.net/2123/1300*.
5. AustLit Database, *http://www.austlit.edu.au/*.
6. For example:

- Ross Coleman, 'Publishing and the digital library – adding value to scholarship and innovation to business', *Learned Publishing*, 22(4) (2009): 297–303. doi:10.1087/20090406.
- Ross Coleman, 'Field, file, data, conference: towards new modes of scholarly publication', *Sustainable Data from Digital Fieldwork. Proceedings of the Conference Held at the University of Sydney*, December 2006. Available at: *http://hdl.handle.net/2123/1300*.
- Rowan Brownlee, 'Research data and repository metadata – policy and technical issues', *Cataloguing & Classification Quarterly*, 47(3/4) (2009). Available at: *http://hdl.handle.net/2123/4996*.
- Sten Christensen, 'Sydney escholarship repository, a case study', *Educause Australasia Conference*, Perth, Western Australia, 3–6 May 2009. Paper No. 99.00 EDUCAUSE. Available at: *http://hdl.handle.net/2123/5027*.
- Creagh Cole, 'Electronic texts at the University of Sydney Library', *Ariadne*, 8 (1997). Available at: *http://www.ariadne.ac.uk/issue8/scholarly-electronic/*.
- Creagh Cole, 'A new continent into literature: the Australian Literature Database at the University of Sydney Library', in *Electronic Publishing '99: Redefining the Information Chain – New Ways and Voices*. Proceedings of an ICCC/IFIP Conference held at the University of Karlskrona/Ronneby, Sweden, 10–12 May 1999, Paper 9909 (Washington, DC: ICCC Press, 1999). Available at: *http://elpub.scix.net/cgi-bin/works/Show?9909*.
- Creagh Cole, 'Form and content: historical and literary texts on the World Wide Web at SETIS'. *http://www.jcu.edu.au/aff/history/articles/cole.htm*.

7. Alison Adams, Stephen Rawles and Alison Saunders, *A Bibliography of French Emblem Books of the Sixteenth and Seventeenth Centuries* (Geneva: Librairie Droz, 1999–2002).
8. ICONCLASS classification scheme. Available at: *http://www.iconclass.nl/*.
9. Stephen Rawles, 'A spine of information headings for emblem-related electronic resources', in *Digital Collections and the*

Management of Knowledge: Renaissance Emblem Literature as a Case Study for the Digitization of Rare Texts and Images. Available at: *http://www.digicult.info/downloads/dc_emblemsbook_lowres.pdf.*

10. Glasgow Emblem Digitisation Project website. Available at: *http://www.ces.arts.gla.ac.uk/html/AHRBProject.htm.*

11. Study and Digitisation of Emblems Project website. Available at: *http://www.italianemblems.arts.gla.ac.uk/index.php* and Alciato at Glasgow Project website, *http://www.emblems.arts.gla.ac.uk/alciato/index.php.*

12. Stephen Rawles, email interview with author, June 2011.

13. Stephen Rawles, email interview with author, June 2011.

14. Open Emblem Portal: *http://media.library.uiuc.edu/projects/oebp/.*

15. HATII website, University of Glasgow: *http://www.gla.ac.uk/departments/hatii/.*

16. Long Room Hub, Trinity College, Dublin: *http://www.tcd.ie/longroomhub/the-institute/about-us/*; M.Phil. in Digital Humanities, Trinity College, Dublin. Available at: *http://www.library.ie/2011/04/29/mphil-in-digital-humanities-and-culture-at-trinity-college-dublin/*; Digital.Humanities@Oxford. Available at: *http://digital.humanities.ox.ac.uk/.*

17. Stephen Rawles, email interview with author, June 2011.

18. Mark Twain Papers and Project. Available at: *http://bancroft.berkeley.edu/MTP/.* Note the current statement of responsibility for the project: 'MTPO is produced by the Mark Twain Papers and Project of the Bancroft Library in collaboration with the University of California Press; the site is hosted by UC Berkeley's Library Systems Office. During 2005–2008 the California Digital Library collaborated in MTPO's creation and initial development.'

19. Lisa Schiff, email interview with author, April 2010.

20. Sharon Goetz, email interview with author, May 2010.

5

Liaison and open access journals

Abstract: Repository Support Officer Jackie Proven at the University of St Andrews Library has used the opportunities provided by the OJS (Open Journal Systems) platform to have useful conversations with faculty and postgraduate students about shaping their proposed open access journals, as well as about open access, repositories and e-scholarship generally. This case study describes how her work with the institutional repository has developed to embrace the additional (though always planned) project of offering OJS functionality to members of the academic community wishing to establish their own journals. With her background in repository support, she recognises this as an important new direction for liaison librarianship and wonders if 'repository people' are in fact becoming the new 'liaison people' rather than the other way round.

Key words: academic liaison, collaboration, digitisation, electronic publishing, e-scholarship, faculty liaison, institutional repository, OJS, open access, Open Journal Systems, scholarly communication.

Jackie Proven took up her post as Repository Support Officer at the University of St Andrews Library in May 2010, bringing with her extensive experience of work in the changing area of scholarly communication from her previous position at the nearby University of Abertay. With a remit to provide operational support for the institutional repository and to ensure its integration with the university's research information system, as well as to establish processes for compliance with funder open access mandates and to set up a pilot service to create online journals, she soon found herself heavily involved in promoting the benefits of the repository and its digital collections generally to potential users throughout the university. The project to establish an open access online journal service has been one which has been particularly well received by the St Andrews academic community, and has led Jackie and Repository Manager Janet Aucock into liaison conversations which have proved fruitful for both Library and Faculty. While the team has reached only the evaluation and trialling stage of the project, it is already clear that St Andrews academics have significant interest in having their open access journals hosted on the Library's OJS platform and that this is an important 'new direction' for the library staff involved.

Although Jackie's appointment was to the Bibliographic Services Division of the Library, from which the Repository is managed, at time of writing (August 2011) discussions are under way to explore the possibility of establishing some degree of integration between the St Andrews Repository and Liaison teams – a change which would recognise the very significant element of liaison activity involved in repository work. This potential development seems to reflect a general trend, with many repository services realising that their core roles of metadata management, data infrastructure organisation and technical support are now being gradually supplemented by a liaison one, their staff exploring and developing the relevant new skills. Jackie herself is conscious of being part of an active and enthusiastic repository community which has a clear sense of mission about what they can offer the academic world. She has certainly been aware of a feeling within that community that it is from within their specialised ranks that the liaison librarians of the future are likely to arise.[1] Like other observers, she feels that 'repository people' are slowly but surely becoming the new 'liaison people.'[2]

Background to the project: the Institutional Repository

In their 2011 article in the *ALISS Quarterly*, Jackie and her manager Janet Aucock describe the various developmental stages through which the St Andrews research repository has passed since its pilot in 2002 and how their work with it has developed to incorporate the new Open Journal Systems service.[3] Crucial to its initial launch was the enthusiasm and persistence of the Deputy Director, Jeremy Upton, who worked hard to secure the resources necessary to get the service off the ground, and who remains a keen advocate of all it can offer. From its primary focus on supporting the deposit of electronic PhD theses in 2006, the repository moved during the 2008 RAE process to establishing links with the university's 'Research Expertise Database', which held metadata for staff research publications. The next stage was the procurement of a new Current Research Information System, with the university implementing PURE in 2010, a system which described all aspects of the university's research activity and provided a workflow for passing full-text research outputs to the repository, now renamed Research@StAndrews:FullText.[4] The exercise is currently in its latest promotional stage, with staff keen to present a joined-up approach to our research community, with coordinated outreach activities. These include joint information sessions (i.e. delivered by both RPO [Research Policy Office] and Library staff) covering REF drivers, the practical benefits of PURE to individual researchers and the opportunities for open access.[5]

Publicising the pilot OJS project is key in this promotional stage, and Jackie and her manager (with additional help from other senior Library staff) have enthusiastically undertaken the task of demonstrating how separately hosted open access journal content can sit alongside the repository's full-text content, giving a wider picture of scholarly activity.

The journals project

The journals project began in response to approaches from academic staff and postgraduates who were interested in creating their own online journals. Content from an Art History journal (*Inferno*) was already held on the repository, and the postgraduate students who edited it were attracted by the idea of transferring it to a bespoke open access platform, where the characteristic look and feel of a print journal could be replicated. The editors of *Theology in Scotland* in the Divinity School were similarly interested, and, as the liaison librarian for that subject area was already a member of the editorial team, this seemed an excellent opportunity for the journal to make the transition from print to electronic form. OJS was identified as a suitable platform, emerging as the front runner for the project on account of its simplicity, flexibility and dependability, and a test site was created to investigate functionality, workflows and appearance. Jackie's reading in the area established that other libraries had found the OJS software reassuringly fit for purpose, the result of

> extensive research into design, reading habits, needs of scholars, editorial flow, and financial costs of online journal hosting that were all considerations when designing and implementing the software. It is the attention paid to these considerations that has helped gain acceptance of the system, and thus contributed to its popularity and growth.[6]

The system supports the full editorial process for journals or more informal publications such as collections of working papers, making provision for all necessary roles (journal manager, editor, copy-editor, proof-reader, reviewer, author, readers) and for the standard workflow through submission, review and editing. It enables flexible open access models – important, as these can change over time – and has a highly configurable set-up process including tips and recommendations. Templates are provided which aid the explicit definition of the scope, policies, author guidelines, and so on for the journal being produced and the system provides history, reporting and statistics. Jackie has found the software straightforward to use, and has appreciated the ease with which changes can be made to the look and feel of the outputs. Images and logos can be added without difficulty, and elements such as footers and navigation links can be introduced, changing the overall theme effectively. Customised style sheets can also be uploaded, ensuring that the journal's look remains consistent.

For the St Andrews project, it was agreed after discussion that the Library would act as the 'electronic distributor' of the journal content, with the School or Department being the publisher. The recommended default policy would be that authors retained copyright, and content would be licensed under Creative Commons. Copyright policies could be amended and would remain under the control of each journal. ISSNs and DOIs would be assigned, and journals would then enjoy the internet benefits of being indexed by Google and other search engines.

Set-up and production stages

Jackie is clear that the pre-set-up liaison conversations with postgraduates and academic staff are crucially important, and recommends that discussions at this stage should establish various parameters. Is there existing content for the journal? How often is publication envisaged? How will users and contributors be managed? Have the journal's scope, editorial policies, author guidelines and copyright issues been discussed? Will there be multiple sections, different formats or supplementary material? An action plan should be drawn up to ensure that suitable infrastructure is in place. Is there an editorial board, and, if so, how does it relate to the academic School? Are there suitable lines of communication with the Library and IT Services, and is it clear who will be doing what? Has a timescale been worked out, as well as projected costs and funding streams, and will there be long-term financial support? Will additional expertise be required for customisation, and will the project be evaluated in due course?

With these considerations in place, Jackie can proceed to the production phase. OJS themselves suggest a tripartite division of labour when setting up a campus-hosted open journal system – there needs to be buy-in from technical staff (server administrator), Library staff and the journal editing team.[7] The first stage is for the Server Administrator to download a free copy of OJS on an existing web server equipped with free PHP language and MySQL database. The software should then be installed using script, enabling the server to upload files, send mail and so on, after which the administrator's role is simply to manage upgrades every six to eight months, and to keep up with regular server security updates. It should be the Librarian's job, say OJS, to advertise the journal, advise potential users on what the system can do, and generate the journal by typing in the title and creating a new user who fills in the details and sets it up. The journal manager then needs to fill in the templates with text, manage submissions, direct reviews and notify users as needed, the whole process culminating in the actual publication of the journal when he or she decides it is ready.

In practice, Jackie has found that things are not quite as clear-cut as this optimum model suggests. Her time is in fact taken up with many other repository-related commitments (deadline-driven work with PURE, REF preparation, discussion of funder mandates with academic staff, and so on), and she is unable to dedicate as much of her working day as might be ideal to the journal project alone. At this pilot stage what the Library is able to offer is a secure server with back-up and preservation, Jackie's time to set up the journal site with basic branding, the digitisation or conversion of archive content and the uploading of back issues, metadata creation, guidance on indexing, accessibility, discovery services, DOIs, etc., plus advice (though not legal advice) on copyright policies and agreements, and about open access business models.[8] Jackie can also offer training for designated people in the journals' editorial teams on how to use the software and configure the OJS functionality, but, where it was initially envisaged that this would be provided once for each journal's staff, leaving them able to proceed with later stages independently, in reality, it was found that staff in the editorial teams change so quickly that time-consuming training has to be offered more or less perpetually. While this is indeed a rounded and effective service as far as it goes, and one clearly run by knowledgeable, enthusiastic and dedicated staff, we are bound to wonder whether additional resource might not increase the capacity and impact of the exercise – we think, for example, of the Canadian York Digital Journals project, which hosts 18 journals on its site.[9] The St Andrews pilot project highlights the constraints implicit in being a very small team, and underlines the difficulties which would be encountered if the service expanded significantly at present staffing levels.

The liaison role

Analysis of the trajectories of Jackie's liaison work is interesting. While she has, of course, liaised importantly with the Faculty and student editors of the two journals now underway, many of her liaison conversations are in fact technical and administrative ones with IT Services staff and with people at the Scottish Digital Libraries Consortium (SDLC), which hosts the university's repository. Again, much of her outreach work is done in conjunction with the Research Policy Office in sessions organised by them to explain to academic staff how to upload their research publications to PURE, and these events have provided a relevant context for both Jackie and Janet to talk about open access issues generally, and the new OJS functionality specifically. Clearly significant alliances are being forged between the Library and RPO staff and the complementariness of their respective functions recognised. Jackie and the Repository Manager see themselves as members not only of the Library Repository Team (which consists of themselves plus a library assistant with day-to-day responsibility for e-theses, all being given a strong steer from the Deputy Director), but also of a wider institutional team incorporating PURE staff, the Library's Bibliometrics Officer, IT staff and members of the Research Policy Office. A complex tracery of inter-departmental connections thus forms the background to their OJS and repository work, the resulting synergy creating useful networks of contacts. Other liaison conversations have been triggered by Jackie's need to speak to Schools, especially the Medical, Science and Social Sciences Schools, about funder mandates for open access publishing. She is responsible for administering the university's Wellcome Trust funding, to which authors can apply to have their open access publishing fees covered, and she finds this a useful 'good news story' to which she can append further information about open access publishing generally, as well as the Library's specific roles in supporting it.

'Actual staff on the ground devoting substantial time to interaction with researchers is crucial,' Jackie writes in her *ALISS* article, interestingly echoing the views of the new advocates of embedded librarianship in her recognition of the need for an essential closeness between the librarian and her research clients.[10] It is clear from her own experiences that setting up OJS journals can indeed provide a context in which such useful closeness can be found and that liaison in this area can produce important outcomes for both sides.

Future plans

Where does she see the service developing in the future? There are possible new directions in the fields of Open Monographs publishing (the repository already holds some material which might be given a fresh new look with this software), and the ePub functionality could be investigated to give the repository's content additional, up-to-date flexibility, making materials compatible with a range of e-readers. The small size of the St Andrews operation is of course a restriction at present, but it is possible that increased academic interest may in future drive change in that area. She would like to see the service gaining a higher profile, stimulating discussion about the possibilities of open access, and hopes that staffing might increase to meet demand. In particular, she feels it would be helpful to have additional dedicated IT and web support for customisation. She is also aware of, and enthusiastic about, the Repository Team's original and longer-term goal of using OJS as a potential teaching tool, perhaps for postgraduates learning about publishing, who could acquire practical experience of reviewing and editing from working with OJS journals.

Jackie has learned a lot from the pilot experience. Interactions with academic staff have confirmed that it's 'not all about pitching something from a library perspective'.[11] Faculty will not 'bite' if they don't like what the Library is offering. She has discovered the sheer, frenetic busyness of the average academic's life and the many conflicting demands on their time which make it difficult to schedule meetings with them, but which also make it imperative that support services step up to the mark to share the load. She has discovered much about their publishing practices, what is important to them, the kinds of relationships they have with publishers and the other work they do, such as editing and peer review. Importantly, she has learned that this is a fruitful area for liaison partnerships between librarians and academics, and is aware that her experience with OJS offers significant pointers to library liaison teams about new directions in which they could usefully develop.

Lessons learned for similar projects

Jackie has found working with OJS has required her not only to know the product in depth, but also to develop the liaison skills necessary to spread the news about it to the academic community. She has acquired both inward-facing knowledge skills as well as outward-facing publicity and marketing ones. She has had to immerse herself in the world of open access, ensuring that she can respond to enquiries about a wide range of related issues, and she has had to learn a lot about academic research activity as it evolves in its twenty-first-century e-scholarship context. Looking after a small-scale OJS project, she advises caution, not wanting to be overwhelmed by demands a still-small team could not meet. Librarians operating in less constrained environments might find themselves able to be less risk-averse and in a position where a high-profile, strongly publicised service might pull in significant business from the academic community. The importance of surveying the market to assess demand is, of course, paramount. This is perhaps an area on which library managers should keep a careful eye, possibly adjusting the service to meet that demand if it increases in due course.

Jackie's advice for librarians proposing to set up open access journals:

- Do loads of homework! You need not only to do thorough testing of OJS functionality, but also to be aware of the range of questions you'll be asked. These might include copyright, resource discovery, indexing services, sources of finance and types of OA models. Make sure you're aware of the norms for publishing in each subject area.

- Be realistic. Keep it small-scale to start with so that you can deliver a quality service, iron out any resource issues and be sure your IT support is adequate. Establish the limits of your service. We have been clear that we are hosting journals as an electronic 'distributor', not a publisher. Be clear about responsibilities and liabilities.

- Convey your enthusiasm! Running this service fits perfectly with our goal to make research outputs more widely available – the Library has a strong commitment to services which support our researchers and promotes research activity in the University. Take every opportunity to discuss scholarly communication and how it is evolving.

Notes

1. Jackie Proven, interview with author, 8 July 2011.
2. e.g. James Toon's OCLC project, *Supporting Research Dissemination*, which aims to examine researcher dissemination behaviours via e.g. institutional repositories, and to use this data to identify new support roles for libraries, in particular for subject liaison librarians. Available at: *http://www.oclc. org/research/activities/desirability/default.htm*. Also, T.O. Walters, 'Reinventing the library: how repositories are causing librarians to rethink their professional roles', *Portal: Libraries and the Academy* 7(2) (2007): 213–25. Available at: *http://smartech.gatech.edu/handle/1853/14421*.
3. Jackie Proven and Janet Aucock, 'Increasing uptake at St Andrews: strategies for developing the research repository', *ALISS Quarterly*, 6(3) (2011): 6–9. Special issue: *Library Services for the 21st Century*.
4. Research@StAndrews:Fulltext, University of St Andrews Institutional Repository, available at: *http://research-repository.st-andrews.ac.uk/*.
5. Proven and Aucock, 'Increasing uptake at St Andrews', op. cit, p. 6.
6. Andrea Kosavic, 'The York Digital Journals Project: strategies for institutional open journal systems implementations', *College and Research Libraries*, 71 (2010): 310.

7. *The Division of Labor on a Campus Hosting Open Journal Systems and Open Conference Systems.* PowerPoint presentation from PKP (Public Knowledge Project). Available at: *http://pkp.sfu.ca/files/Division%20of%20Labor.pdf*.

8. Jackie has found the SURF Copyright Toolbox invaluable (Available at: *http://copyrighttoolbox.surf.nl/copyrighttoolbox/*) and frequently refers enquirers to it. Another useful guide is available at: *http://www.doaj.org/bpguide/plan/*.

9. Kosavic, 'The York Digital Journals Project', op. cit, pp. 310–21.

10. Proven and Aucock, 'Increasing uptake at St Andrews', op. cit., p. 8. For commentary on embedded librarianship, see the Conclusion.

11. Jackie Proven, email interview with author, July 2011.

6

Liaison and community outreach: a Friends of the Library group

Abstract: At the University of St Andrews Library Alice Crawford decided to try to address her library's image problem by setting up a Friends of the Library group. The Library, she felt, needed to be re-established in people's minds as a strong, refreshed and exciting *research* institution, and a Friends group with a remit to promote the library's reputation and encourage interest in its collections might go some way towards rehabilitating this patient with a difficult past. The case study describes the various stages of the venture, from drafting a constitution to establishing a Committee, designing a web page, organising visits to interesting libraries and running a series of well-attended twice-yearly lectures. The project has provided Alice with liaison opportunities outside her normal sphere of library activities, and she has enjoyed being able to draw the recovering library to people's attention. The Friends, and the King James Library Lectures which she has also run, have been a subtle and unusual marketing venture as well as a new and interesting direction for her liaison work.

Key words: academic liaison, faculty liaison, Friends of the Library, King James Library Lectures, liaison, librarians, librarianship, marketing, outreach, roles.

On taking up my post of Academic Liaison Librarian for Arts and Divinity at the University of St Andrews in January

2007, I realised that two particular challenges presented by my job description would be to 'develop strategy and provide services relevant to the research needs of the University', and to 'find new ways to communicate with customers and promote Library resources'.

The situation was complicated by the fact that I had joined a library which was in the process of recovering from long years of underinvestment and understaffing. It had earned a reputation during that time as an institution struggling to meet the needs of students and staff. Answers to the 2007 Student Satisfaction Survey indicated the users' clear perception that all was not well, and that change was urgently needed.

This was a library with an image problem. However ardently and energetically staff worked to address matters at a practical level – securing increased budgets, flooding the shelves with new stock, appointing new personnel, pushing forward with plans for a massive redevelopment of the building – the difficulty of convincing the academic community that the changes were good remained insuperable. Disappointment with – even hostility towards – the Library had become deeply ingrained in its customers, lack of respect towards its staff endemic. With my liaison remit of strategic development and resource promotion responsibilities, it seemed to me that this was an issue with which I could usefully engage and attempt to make a difference. While other members of the academic liaison team investigated new ways of communicating with undergraduate customers via Web 2.0 technology – opening library Facebook pages, introducing a Meebo enquiry service, establishing a library presence in Second Life – I decided to think outside the Web 2.0 box and explore the possibilities of different types of communication with different types of customer.

As someone who had used libraries to conduct my own academic research, I felt that the heart of the problem lay in the fact that too many of the Library's users thought of it as simply a large concrete box housing textbooks for students. Undergraduates were dissatisfied with it because they thought there were never enough copies of these textbooks available when they wanted them (the day before the essay was due) and academic staff were dissatisfied with it because it was not a St Andrews-by-the-sea version of the Bodleian, delivering research collections and services appropriate to the University's sub-Oxbridge image. The Library, it seemed to me, needed to be re-established in people's minds as a strong, refreshed and exciting *research* institution. If the academic community could be convinced that the Library was serious about synchronising its collections policies with the aspirations of a research-intensive university, and that those collections were being competently managed by staff who understood the nature of that research – its value and urgency – then a significant step would have been taken towards reclaiming the Library's damaged image. While staff and research students would probably be the first to be impressed by this gradual restoration of the Library's reputation, an eventual cascade effect on undergraduates would be likely to follow. It was possible that they would, in time, see themselves studying in and having at their disposal, a library housing respected research collections, as well as the multiple copies of textbooks they so vigorously demanded. The knee-jerk instinct to criticise would be checked and they might – though this could take several student generations to become apparent – learn to respond more thoughtfully and more positively to student satisfaction questionnaires eliciting their responses to library services.

How, then, to revitalise the Library's image by re-associating it with the university's research mission? Clearly the Special

Collections department was already playing an important role in this by promoting its rare book and manuscript material through extensive and much appreciated teaching programmes targeting History, English and Modern Languages postgraduates. Clearly, too, much was being done at an administrative level via the Director's work on the new Strategic Planning Document for the Library, which placed a determined new emphasis on the 'provision of services and resources to support the research ambitions' of the university as the Unit's first strategic priority. There did seem to be a role here too, however, for Academic Liaison to boost and supplement these initiatives. Why not, I wondered, extend my liaison activities beyond the usual conversations with library representatives and students about reading lists and information literacy classes, and start some conversations with a wider circle of library users? Why not set up a Friends of the Library group, such as I had seen in action at other university libraries, and see what could be done to 'rehabilitate' the Library as a research-focused place of interest to users outside the university campus?

Setting up the group

A supportive Director, who had also seen a Friends of the Library group work well elsewhere, gave the go ahead, and I was quickly given the task of devising a Constitution and setting up a committee. The University's Development Office was very helpful in providing constitution guidelines for alumni groups, and it proved fairly straightforward to convert this into a draft constitution for the potential Friends. It seemed important to have this in place before calling a meeting of the group so that basic parameters could be established, and I found it helpful to clarify my thoughts on the group's aims for this document. These eventually resolved themselves into the following:

- To promote the reputation of the Library and encourage interest in its collections.

- To promote and facilitate the learning and research mission of the University Library via the organisation of scholarly activities.

- To engage with local, national and international academic and lay communities in the work and mission of the University Library, particularly Special Collections.

- To support the Library in its acquisition of, preservation of, and provision of access to rare books, manuscripts, collections of papers and photographs and other rare and/ or valuable items which it could not normally afford.

- To act as a channel for gifts of books and manuscripts to enhance the Library's collections, especially those of the Special Collections Department.

The creation of a Friends web-page on the Library site was the next stage in willing the group into existence, after which there followed the fun of inviting people to serve on the Friends committee.[1] The Director and I agreed that this should consist of a Chairperson, a Vice-Chairperson, an Honorary Secretary, an Honorary Treasurer and about ten other members, and that the Director of Library Services, the Head of Special Collections, the Academic Liaison Librarian for Arts and Divinity and one other member of Library staff should be ex officio members. Members would be elected for a period of three years, after which they would be eligible for re-election. In selecting people to invite to the Committee, the criterion used was basically 'Who would be interested?' We approached two current and two recently retired senior academics known to be enthusiastic library users, a member of the University Court, two members of staff from the National Library of Scotland and two retired members of our own Library staff. We were delighted when Professor Kay Redfield Jamison from Johns Hopkins University accepted our invitation to be Chairperson. Known to us as an Honorary Professor in the St Andrews School of English, the eclectic span of her interests across both the Sciences and the Arts made her the perfect person to head up the group and to suggest in doing so the continuing relevance of libraries to both areas. This international element in the Committee would be particularly helpful, we felt, not only in raising the profile of the group but also in allowing us to hear at first hand about North American fundraising trends and practices.

The Committee met for the first time on 1 June 2007, and, having endorsed the draft Constitution and decided on subscription levels, set about arranging a membership drive and a programme of activities. I undertook the onerous task of organising a mailshot to town and gown sources, publicising the existence of the new group and inviting people to join. All academic and academic-related members of the university staff received a printed leaflet and application form, as did 50 or so non-university readers identified as dedicated users of the Special Collections Department. I also arranged for articles and photographs to appear in the university's staff magazine *The StAndard*, alumnus publications *FourteenTen* and *The Alumnus Chronicle* as well as in local publications *The St Andrews Citizen* and *St Andrews in Focus*. The Reprographics Department produced an eyecatchingly colourful banner, which was displayed in the Library's main reading room where students were routed to have their graduation photographs taken – it was hoped that this would be a useful point of contact with new alumni and their parents, and that students might think at that stage of signing up to maintain a link with the library of their *alma mater*.

The response was interesting and on the whole encouraging. By the end of the Friends' first year of existence around 45 people had taken out life membership of £150, and a further six had committed to an annual subscription at £30. Total membership has now risen to 65 in July 2011. I was slightly surprised at the very low uptake from current members of academic staff. The massive initial mailing elicited returns from only six academics outside those elected to the Committee. One student and one member of the Principal's office signed up, and there was no response at all from any of the new alumni so hopefully propositioned at the graduation photograph hall. The uptake was very definitely from interested, bookish 'town' and retired but lively 'gown' – people, in other words, with time to spare for the activities so temptingly displayed (we hoped) in the publicity material.

Programme of events

Rolling out a programme of events has been a most enjoyable and rewarding aspect of the project. The Committee felt that a mixture of lectures, visits and treasure tours of Special Collections should be offered, and encouraged suggestions from the membership about what they would like to see featured in the schedule. Our inaugural lecture was delivered by Ronald Milne, Director of Scholarship and Collections at the British Library, who spoke on 'Research Libraries in the Digital Age', and this was followed later in the group's first year by 'Writing Scotland's Photography' by Dr Tom Normand of the University's School of Art History. This pattern of maintaining a mixture of national and local speakers in the programme has seemed to be important and to work well, enabling the Library both to display the strengths of its own (for example, world-class photography) collections and to demonstrate its place as a well-networked player in the wider library world. In Autumn 2008, Dr Gillian Dow of the University of Southampton spoke impressively about the reading material found by early women writers in 'Their Fathers' Libraries', drawing on the rich resources of Chawton House Library, and in Spring 2009 Dr Sarah Thomas of the Bodleian Library swept us into an enthusiastic consideration of the possibilities for new library buildings in her talk, 'Creating Space or Creative Space: Planning Tomorrow's Library Today'. Other speakers have included Professor Andrew Murphy, who explored the Library's Shakespeare collections in his provocatively titled lecture, 'Shakespeare at St Andrews', and Faith Liddell, who drew on her experiences as Director of Festivals Edinburgh to speak on 'Books Vision and Ambition in an Age of Austerity'.

Audiences for all lectures so far have been excellent – rooms have been booked for 90 people in each case and have been comfortably filled. Considerable effort goes into the advance publicity. Posters are displayed in all Schools within the University as well as in prominent places throughout the town, hand-delivered by our faithful secretary, who recognises that face-to-face contact with noticeboard organisers produces better results. The event is submitted to the university's News web pages and given coverage there, and an advertisement is always sent to the local newspaper, making it clear that the lecture is open to all, not just subscribing members of the Friends. Copy and accompanying photographs are sent to local newspapers after the event, and articles sometimes appear recording the occasion. Emails targeting particular potential audiences are also sent out shortly before each lecture, for example, to English, History and Art History postgraduates and members of staff who might be interested in a particular topic. Post-lecture refreshments seem to be much appreciated, and form an integral part of the evening – a wine and canapés reception followed the inaugural lecture, with tea and coffee satisfying audiences after subsequent talks. The opportunity to chat is much appreciated, and I have been conscious of facilitating a useful and enjoyable new forum for liaison with a new tranche of library users.

While lectures have always been scheduled for 5.15pm on weekdays to enable staff to attend after work, it was recognised that there was a need for other events at other times. The group has now also enjoyed a 'treasures tour' of Special Collections, a guided visit to the University's new museum (MUSA), and a wonderfully engrossing Saturday afternoon among the incunabula and other rare books of a local great house library. More 'further afield' outings are planned, and these are seen to be valuable as occasions on which the Friends can be drawn together socially as a group of people indulging a shared interest in libraries.

Finance and administration

Administratively and financially the group is slightly problematic. The preponderance of life members, who have taken advantage of the generous opening offer of a single one-off payment of £150, means that the Friends' finances are currently and for the foreseeable future static. Ongoing income from the half-dozen annual members is negligible, and this is an issue which is about to be addressed by a newly established subcommittee. They will need to explore possibilities for extending the membership (which could be difficult in that the pool of interested subscribers may already have been exhausted), and think of new ways of generating income. If the group is to fulfil its remit of supporting the Library in its acquisition of rare books or manuscripts, it will need to ensure that the pot of its finances refills regularly after taking the 'hit' of subsidising purchases. There is, too, the fact that any fundraising activities will need to be carefully choreographed with the University's Development Office, which is simultaneously liaising with potential donors over a major library redevelopment project, scheduled for 2011–2013. I have found myself engaged in interesting liaison conversations with Development staff over the scope of the Friends' remit, the group's charity status and approaches to potential supporters. Discussions have always been positive and helpful, but have underlined the fact that the Friends exist in a slightly vulnerable limbo between town and gown, governed by university regulations but strongly shaped by the requirements of a non-university membership.

A second subcommittee produces the Friends' Newsletter, which appears twice a year and is billed as one of the benefits of membership. This glossy, four-page publication contains reports of Friends' events, news of forthcoming ones and short articles on rare book or manuscript topics. Driven largely by Special Collections preoccupations and staff, the Winter 2008/9 edition contains an item on marginalia in some of the Library's eighteenth-century texts, an account of a local researcher's work to transcribe a manuscript Civil War diary for publication, an introduction to the new Photographic Archivist and his work developing and curating the Library's historic photography collections, plus a report of the Friends' autumn lecture by Dr Gillian Dow. Liaison with the Reprographics department has resulted in an attractive design featuring the Friends' distinctive masthead and logo. In the early stages of its existence, the group fought a courteous battle with the External Affairs Office for permission to call itself the 'Friends of St Andrews University Library' rather than the tongue-twistingly difficult but politically correct 'Friends of the University of St Andrews Library'. In the end, quiet insistence paid off, and the neat short version of the name heads a news-sheet stylistically positioned between town and gown, touching base neatly with the Library's many other publications, while maintaining its own character and tone.

The Friends seem now to have 'taken off' and to be enjoying a happy existence, semi-independently of the Library. I continue to supply some administrative support, booking rooms and teas and nudging along the lecture programme with ideas for speakers and making arrangements for their accommodation and remuneration. The honorary secretary, however, takes on the more onerous responsibilities of producing minutes, agendas and other paperwork, and it is good to see this 'baby bird' of a group spreading its wings and beginning to fly the nest.

King James Library Lectures

Encouraged by the Friends' success, and inspired by the plans being put in place by the university for celebrating its 600th anniversary in 2013, I have now launched an even more ambitious 'companion' lecture programme, this time on the theme of 'The Meaning of the Library'.[2] The King James Library Lecture Series takes its name from the University's oldest reading room, the King James Library, established in 1612 by a bequest from King James VI and I of Scotland, and described by Dr Johnson as an 'elegant and luminous bookroom'. The aim of the series is to try to articulate what the library as an institution has meant to different generations of society throughout history, and to offer some visions of what it might become in our own day and in the future. Working in discussion with academics, I

101

have extended invitations to a range of internationally renowned figures in the academic and library worlds, asking them to deliver lectures on Ancient, Medieval, Renaissance, Enlightenment, Victorian and contemporary libraries, as well as on Libraries in Film and Libraries in Fiction. The Library Directorate has again been immensely helpful towards this project, and provided a generous budget which has enabled me to offer substantial, and I hope attractive, speaker fees. We were honoured to have our inaugural lecture delivered by Dr James Billington, Librarian of Congress, in June 2009, who spoke eloquently on 'The Modern Library and Global Democracy'. Professor Andrew Pettegree delivered an excellent talk on 'The Renaissance Library and the Challenge of Print' in November 2009, and Dr Stephen Enniss of the Folger Shakespeare Library fascinated his audience in March 2010 with his reflections on his experiences in building a contemporary manuscripts collection at the University of Emory – 'Casting and Gathering: Libraries, Archives and the Modern Writer'. Harvard's Professor Robert Darnton drew another appreciative audience in June 2010 with his lecture on Libraries of the Enlightenment, as did Professor Laura Marcus in April 2011 with 'The Library in Film' and Professor Richard Gameson in October 2011 with 'The Image of the Medieval Library.' Future lecturers are scheduled to include Professor Edith Hall on Libraries in the Ancient World and Professor Marina Warner on Libraries in Fiction. There is a plan to collect all the lectures into a book entitled *The Meaning of the Library*, to be published in 2013, and launched as part of the 600th anniversary celebrations that year.

The project has again afforded me liaison opportunities outside the normal spheres of library activities. Personal printed invitations to the lectures are sent to a wide range of university staff, and I have welcomed this chance to draw the Library to people's attention. The theme itself seems to interest people, and it is reassuring to see the lecture theatres filled with audiences prepared to devote an hour of their day to thinking about the value of libraries. It is good, too, to be able to offer the academic community world-class speakers, and an intellectually stimulating series of talks, rather than simply the run-of-the-mill information bulletins which normally emanate from the Library – it is restorative both for the Library's image and for its staff's morale to be associated with the high-quality thought which the lectures embody. Sending out invitations to the Librarian of Congress's lecture to the Directors of all the other Scottish University Libraries, and to the Director of the National Library of Scotland, I had an invigorating sense of putting the University of St Andrews Library on the map.

My experiences with these two lecture series have shown me how well placed a liaison librarian can be to contribute to the marketing and communication activities of her library. Marketing academic libraries is not always about handing out free pens and mouse-mats to undergraduates in Orientation Week. There are important markets beyond the obvious undergraduate one, and it may require subtler, and more intellectually strenuous, efforts to convince the wider academic research community that the Library is indeed on its wavelength, its staff qualified to understand their information needs. The subtext to both lecture series is an attempt to restore our Library's intellectual credibility – by bringing bright people to talk, and by providing space from time to time in which ideas about libraries and their collections can be thought about, we hope to convince our various constituencies that we are bright people too, and can be trusted to provide a service of value to them. It is a gentler, more sophisticated liaison activity, and one which in our own case is so far proving well worthwhile.

Lessons learned for similar projects

As with all such projects, knowing one's market before proceeding is always key. I had worked at the university long enough to be aware of potential interest in a Friends group among recently retired members of academic staff and among regular users of the Library's Special Collections. I had also lived in the town long enough to know that this was an area rich with societies for the intellectually interested, and that there was room for one for townspeople inclined to support the University Library. I was aware from the beginning that this was likely to be a 'club' for older people, and that it probably would not appeal to undergraduate students. Current academics too were likely to be too busy to play any very active part, however supportive of the library they might feel. Marketing the group to the targeted constituencies where interest had been observed allowed it a secure launch-pad in fruitful territory.

It is important too, I found, always to keep the group's longer-term future in mind. Care is needed to keep its finances viable. The *raison d'être* of the group, the provision of support for the Special Collections Department and the Library generally, has to inform all its activities. The activities themselves must ensure that the coffers are continually replenished so that this support can be offered – money has to be available, for instance, to help the Library buy the rare book or precious manuscript it would not normally be able to afford.

The group's prospectus of activities needs to be kept fresh and interesting. For me, it was sometimes difficult to come up with new ideas for speakers and visits, and, although members were encouraged to put forward suggestions, the burden of doing so and of making the arrangements in reality usually fell on me. It would be better to have a committee of people constantly tasked with maintaining the programme of activities and sharing a richer variety of ideas. It would be more efficient, too, to share the administrative tasks where possible.

Needless to say, it is important that members enjoy the activities – lectures, outings and so on – whether these are transparently for fund-raising or not. A group that has fun together and looks forward to meetings is likely to work well together towards any more worthy goal it is set.

Advice for anyone proposing to set up a Friends of the Library group or related lecture programme:

- Liaise with members to discover the names of people they would like to hear lecture – think of what *they* would like to hear about, not you!

- Ensure you have a decent budget in place – lecture fees, accommodation, travel expenses for speakers and catering for large audiences don't come cheap.

- Think in terms of creating a 'cultural programme' with a variety of activities in addition to lectures – make each event high profile, with good publicity, and of course always include food!

Notes

1. Friends of St Andrews University Library website, *http://www. st-andrews.ac.uk/library/friends/*.
2. King James Library Lectures website, *http://www.st-andrews. ac.uk/library/news/lectures/*.

7

Liaison and library buildings

Abstract: Librarian of Girton College, Cambridge, Frances Gandy, demonstrates the critical importance of liaison skills in the project management and design of a new library building. Bringing the Duke Library Building to fruition in 2005 involved her in liaison conversations not only with academic, administrative and library staff, but also with architects, finance committees, fundraisers, donors, alumni and the builders themselves. This case study explores her experience and showcases the ways in which her significant liaison and organisational skills have worked together to achieve a superbly pleasing library building which has the distinction of being essentially designed by librarians.

Key words: academic liaison, faculty liaison, fundraising, librarians, librarianship, library architecture, library buildings, library design, project management, SCONUL.

If a case study is needed to demonstrate the impressive multiple skills of professional librarians suddenly called to project manage the design and delivery of new library buildings, no better exemplar can be found than that of Frances Gandy and the development of the new Duke Building of Girton College, Cambridge, opened in April 2005.

This is a project in which 'academic liaison' must be interpreted in its widest and most meaningful sense. None of the library staff involved was designated a 'liaison librarian' in contractual or job-description terms, yet all – and particularly the Librarian herself – found themselves liaising in critically important ways with the challengingly wide range of constituencies and stakeholders the project touched. There was liaison with architects, with finance committees, with fundraisers and donors, with academic, administrative and internal library staff, with current and former students, and with contractors both on and off-site during the eventual stressful months of 'having the builders in'. As Project Co-ordinator, the Librarian's task was to orchestrate multiple conversations and to ensure that this liaison produced results.

Designed by architects Allies & Morrison, the Duke Building received a national RIBA Award in 2006, as well as a Civic Trust Award and the SCONUL Library Design Award (smaller buildings) in 2007.[1] A text-book study for architects in how to create the small but perfect library building, its story should also demonstrate to librarians how their meaningful liaison with design and technical professionals can result in a building which delights and satisfies both its creators and its users.[2]

Background to the project

Librarian Frances Gandy emphasises how from the very start the building was designed 'from the inside out'.[3] Conversations between herself and the architect were key from the outset, the focus always on the need to translate library requirements into practical, deliverable realities:

> For example, we needed good sight-lines between areas in order to minimise the need for staff, since we had agreed that we would not increase the staff establishment. We needed flexible space that could be changed in future

if needs changed or emphases in service and provision were altered. We wanted a sense of all activities being integrated and interdependent, so transparency and physical connection were important. The building was thus designed from the inside outwards.[4]

The need for a new building had been established as far back as 1996, when the Librarian had submitted to the College Council a proposal for an extension to the existing building. New accommodation was required for the College's archival collections and special collections of books. The existing archive was in a single-storey building under a leaking flat roof, and was rapidly running out of space. Current standards for conservation and environmental control were not being met, and there was no separate space for researchers working in the archive itself. In these cramped conditions, there were no proper facilities for the conservation of materials, and no reading room for users of the special collections books, which were 'scattered variously around the college'.[5] IT resource space was limited to what could be squeezed in between the stacks, and this area was in urgent need of expansion. New offices were also badly needed for staff, who were struggling with insufficient space for book processing and administrative functions, and the lack of cloakroom facilities for both staff and students was becoming an increasing problem. The need for a small staff kitchen was also itemised.

In response to this proposal for an extension, the College initially appointed architects to conduct a feasibility study and some estimates of costs. The Library was staffed at the time by the Librarian, an Archivist, an Assistant Librarian and two library assistants. Of this group, the Librarian and the Archivist worked closely with the architects to develop a brief which offered practical solutions to the building's various problems and would ensure the smooth functioning of its inter-related departments. The design process was then suspended for a time while fundraising took place (more of this below), but once the majority of the funds were assured, and the College had authorised the building process to proceed, a subcommittee of the College's Buildings Committee was formed to steer the project. This Project Subcommittee met monthly and was chaired by the Mistress of the College, and included the Bursar, the Librarian and the Development Director. An external Project Manager was appointed from Arup Project Management to ensure that the building came in on time and on budget. He drew up schedules and guidelines for the design team and contractors, and attended regular meetings with them. He also attended the monthly Project Subcommittee meetings and produced a monthly report. The Librarian was appointed as Project Co-ordinator and as such acted as the interface between the design team, the contractors and the College. Once the building work started, she conducted a site visit every day and maintained the site diary.

Project development

The strong collaborative relationship between the Library and the architects continued to thrive throughout the working up of the design. To the original brief were added the strict standards of conservation and environment, in particular adherence to BS5454:2000, and the requirement to achieve as far as possible a low energy use. Crucially, too, the input of professional departmental managers from both the Library and Archive areas ensured the design took into account the future direction of academic library provision and the optimum standards for archival practice. Frances Gandy confirms:

> We were consulted on almost every detail and design
> decision and were able to influence choices at every
> level and throughout the process, even down to location
> and quantity of power points, Ethernet points, and the
> furniture . . .[6]

The Librarian reported back to the Project Subcommittee, but the College gave her a generous degree of discretion and responsibility to negotiate and make decisions – a factor which has been important in determining the Library's sense of 'owning' the project as a whole. In terms of aesthetics, the conversations between the Library and the architects were also significant. The Library wished to achieve a balance between old and new, and to maintain a 'courteous relationship' between the proposed modern extension and the older neighbouring section, designed by the third generation of the Waterhouse family with Giles Gilbert Scott. Naturally this involved attention to scale and to materials, and frequent meetings were held in Cambridge and London between the architects and the Librarian to ensure these details were attended to. The Librarian also worked with the architects in helping to present elements of the proposed design to various organisations which might strengthen their case to the planners, e.g. the Royal Fine Art Commission and the local Parish Council. The experiences of other libraries were taken into account, and visits were made to Churchill College Archive Centre to look at their rolling stacks and conservation room fit-outs. Phone calls were made to a range of professional colleagues to ask about their experiences of certain products and companies, and consultations with various individuals, including Dr Christopher Kitching, former Director of the National Archives, proved invaluable.

The liaison role

In addition to liaising with the architects, the Librarian was strongly aware of the need to maintain good communication about the project with various constituencies within the College itself, to ensure that the building was developing along lines they approved of, and to keep them informed of developments. Within the College's relatively democratic infrastructure, all elements of the community are represented on its executive. The College Council, the key executive committee, includes elected members of the Fellowship and also elected members from the graduate and undergraduate communities. All members of the community, therefore, have a say in decision-making. Issues about buildings are always referred to the Augmented Council, which includes the entire fellowship, thus giving another, even broader, forum for discussion. In relation to this particular project, the College arranged for the design team to present their ideas to the Fellowship in a series of special presentations. These focused primarily on the sensitive issues of the exterior appearance of the building and its impact on the much-loved front elevation of the College, and the engineering and structural issues relating to the environmental strategy. At these sessions Fellows were able to put questions to the design team and discuss the viability of various options.

Care was taken, too, to liaise with alumni. Although there was no formal consultation process with them, a number of public relations exercises were undertaken to reassure them that nothing detrimental to their beloved buildings was being planned. The upper reading room of the existing library was particularly cherished, and the Librarian and others in the team were at pains to ensure that this was not touched in any way, and that views of the new building from its windows would be congenial. Thus the flat roof of one new section is planted with sedum, and the other flat roof is laid with hand-beaten lead panels.

Internal liaison with the College's library staff was, of course, a crucial, ongoing activity. The Librarian reported back to them regularly from the Project Subcommittee, ensuring that they knew what was happening at each stage. Both managers and library assistants were consulted about their own workspaces, and reassured that what they felt was important in the new building was being taken into account. Concerns or suggestions were fed back into the plans. Regular 'don't panic' meetings were held so that all staff were aware of timetables and schedules, and these helped give a sense of control and structure. Project-related responsibilities were charted, colour-coded and distributed among relevant staff as necessary, though many of these involved other College departments, e.g. electricians for temporary power and light supplies, the Computer Office for rigging up and networking computers for temporary offices, House Services for moving furniture and the Maintenance Department for sundry miscellaneous jobs. At management level, the Archivist contributed significantly to the task by researching the fine detail required for environmental control parameters, recommended conservation standard fittings and equipment, lux levels and the like, while the Assistant Librarian was masterful at updating and keeping tabs on all the administrative fine-tuning required to keep the library functioning while operation centres moved around. As Project Co-ordinator the Librarian found this support invaluable, as she could rely on both managers to supply her with the detailed information needed for strategic decisions. She was also highly appreciative of her staff's commitment to keeping the library service going under pressure.

During the noisy, messy stage during which the actual building work was done, staff coped well with the many pressures. The building work had to be phased to offer the least disruption to students during exam time, and operations began on the site immediately after the exams finished in June 2003. At the end of the project, the builders were effectively clear of the site just one week before the start of the Michaelmas term of 2004, allowing only a few days to relocate office and ensure services could be resumed in time for the return of staff and students. Access to collections was restricted for the minimum time possible, since delays would have had huge implications for the College's educational operations. Some book collections were made inaccessible for a brief period over two summers, and the archival collections were moved off-site for over a year to avoid any risk of damage. This meant that there was no possibility of archive research during that time, though basic enquiries were answered.

Library assistants and the Assistant Librarian were moved during the building phase to the upper floor of the existing library, and a temporary office was established to incorporate everything they required for effective operations, including networked computers. A separate entrance to this area was established so that there was no need for staff to be involved in the building site section, and they were also well away from dust. The book stacks of the lower library were sealed up with plastic, and became part of the building site and thus a no-go area for staff. The Archivist was given an adjacent student room from which to work, and in which she could house a few key items from the archival collections with which she could deal with basic enquiries and continue to work on various projects. The archive and special collections areas were not complete when the building opened to students in October 2004, so the Archivist was temporarily housed in the Librarian's office, and took the Librarian's work space.

Fundraising

In this project the Librarian was heavily involved in fundraising activities. Once the early feasibility study was completed, the College decided that the money for the new building ought to be raised before it would commit itself finally to the building going ahead. As the College at that time did not have its development operations fully functioning, the onus of fundraising therefore fell on a group of individuals including the Librarian and the Archivist. The Mistress of Girton was a strong supporter of the project and set up a Campaign Committee comprising a core team of around eight alumni, the Librarian, the Archivist and later the Development Director, under the chairmanship of the Mistress. The group held regular meetings in London and Cambridge, and co-opted a number of other experts from time to time for special advice on events and mailings. The responsibility for initiating and preparing funding applications, however, fell on the shoulders of the Librarian until the latter stages of the campaign when, following restructuring in the Development Office, the Development Director took a more active role.

The first major fundraising bid was an application to the Heritage Lottery Fund. This was co-ordinated by the Librarian, and partly written by her and the Archivist in conjunction with the architects, who also produced the final application brochure. Unfortunately the bid was unsuccessful, and the Campaign Committee therefore had to return to the College and ask permission to continue funding by other means.

A huge campaign was mounted to reach out to alumni, and the bulk of the project funds came in the end from this source. Girton has the highest ratio of alumni donors among the Cambridge colleges, and there is no doubt in the Librarian's mind that for many the idea of raising money for a building which would properly look after and conserve the College's history appealed to the imaginations of alumni, who were understandably proud of their College's heritage. The first residential college for the higher education of women in England, Girton has always had a library which featured importantly in its history, as well as a strong tradition of donor help. When it was first established, a call went out for donations of books from its supporters, and as a consequence copies of their own work came from William Morris, the Darwins, John Ruskin, George Eliot and others. Whole libraries were also donated in the early years, such as Mary Somerville's scientific library and Helen Blackburn's collection of books on women's campaigns for the recognition of their rights in society, e.g. in industry, law, politics and education. In this new, twenty-first-century campaign, alumni responded generously to appeals, and hundreds of gifts were received, ranging from modest sums to donations of several thousand pounds. A student-staffed telethon raised considerable amounts in phone conversations with former students. Carefully briefed in all areas of the project, they talked many alumni through the scheme and acted as impressive ambassadors for the venture. Some donors asked for their gifts to be targeted to specific areas, and these requests were accommodated. Those, for example, who felt that the primary purpose of the College was to educate the current generation, and that fundraising should be focused on that, were shown the expanded and spacious IT Resources area, and how that fitted into the recommended model of HE library provision in the twenty-first century. Staff offices were also, indirectly, part of that provision, in so far as adequately-housed staff would now be able to offer the professional information services which members of College require. It was also emphasised that the research resources held in the archive and special collections would now be securely housed and fully available to students for use in their dissertations.

Other funds came from sources such as organisations or companies connected with Girton's history, and applications – usually written by the Librarian – were also made to many charitable organisations in the UK and the United States. The Librarian and Archivist mounted several special promotional exhibitions and delivered a series of promotional talks in venues which ranged from the House of Lords to Queen's College, Harley St. In the final stages of the project, as part of the process in which the Development Office was restructured, a team of fundraising consultants was brought in to advise on both this campaign and College fundraising generally, but it seems clear that the bulk of the fundraising work had by this time been successfully managed by the Librarian.

Library involvement in the design

Overall, the singular success of this project appears to have been in large part attributable to the very close engagement of the Librarian and her staff with the design, architectural, technical and financial teams tasked with bringing the building to fruition. Her informed, sympathetic liaison with the many disparate groups, each with its own essential input to the project, confirmed the vital role she played as Co-ordinator, and ultimately ensured that the Library achieved a successful result. In the Client Comment document she wrote for the SCONUL Awards Panel, Frances Gandy sings the building's praises two years after it opened.[7] 'The new Duke Building delivers what we had hoped for in terms of both its aesthetic and its functional character,' she affirms. 'As clients we have been closely involved in both the design and construction phases, but find our expectations of the quality of the working space to have been exceeded.' She is delighted by the fact that 'this spacious and light working environment has attracted significantly more students and fellows into the library than hitherto', and that the connections established between the existing book stacks and the new IT area work well, allowing readers to move seamlessly between the two as twenty-first-century patterns of working demand. She is satisfied that the building is adaptable and flexible for future use. A hollow floor allows all services to run within the cavity, and, with the floor constructed of removable panels, the number of data points can easily be increased in future. The new staff areas provide a 'calming and high quality working environment', and the Archives area is newly conformant to the standards of BS5454:2000. The building is energy-efficient, a combination of thermal mass, earth ducts and small AHUs reducing energy consumption by approximately 50 per cent. Above all, both readers and library staff love the space which has been produced. Researchers praise the high quality of the Littler Reading Room's design, and library staff enjoy the clever use of glass partitions and internal windows which allow them to maintain clear sight-lines from one work section to another. A gratifying number of College staff and alumni have commented that the new building has drawn their attention to aspects of the old that they had not previously noticed or appreciated, the result, the Librarian feels, of the architects' understanding of and respect for the existing buildings and their history.

As an example of a library essentially designed by librarians, Girton College's Duke Building is surely unsurpassed. It is a superb demonstration of what can be achieved when librarians branch out from their traditional roles and embrace the new skills which a new situation demands. As Librarian and Project Co-ordinator, Frances Gandy confirms that she gained a great deal of satisfaction from what was an enormously creative process. She learned a lot, she says, about project management and co-ordination, as well as huge amounts about the process and intricacies of all aspects of building projects. She can also recite elements of BS5454:2000 off by heart! Her staff, too, learned a great deal about running and co-ordinating a multi-faceted project, and how to offer a quality library service under duress. The process, they say, strengthened their ability to work as a team, a valuable by-product of the exercise. Beyond all, however, the best outcome was the end result of the building itself, which continues to give them all huge pleasure when they walk into it every morning.

Lessons learned for similar projects

The Girton Library project has clearly been an exhausting but hugely rewarding one for those involved. The case study makes clear the vital importance of careful preparation. Those who are going to use the building must take time to specify their needs in detail, to think about service developments which the building might have to accommodate in the longer term, and inform themselves about the relevant standards and specifications to which the work needs to be carried out. They need to read up on this new subject that will affect them and their work so closely, and to be aware of similar projects elsewhere.

The study highlights, too, how the Project Co-ordinator, positioned in the library, must both think and act strategically, positioning herself where her voice can be heard and ensuring that she has sufficient executive authority to carry decisions through to fruition. She must bring to the job a remarkable skill set which includes managerial prowess, organisational exactitude, architectural vision, awareness of client needs, diplomacy, good judgement, enthusiasm, courage, sensitivity and, perhaps above all, perseverance.

Advice from Frances Gandy for librarians proposing to embark on a library building project:

- Before you say a word to anyone, do your homework and map out your infrastructure. Decide on your goals. Research the standards that you wish to attain and work out the connectivity of your operations. Read the professional literature and future-proof your plans. Build in flexibility. Go for the best and don't take 'no' for an answer.

- Ensure that you position yourself strategically, with sufficient political clout within your organisation to influence decisions, both in the planning and throughout the design and building processes. Ideally you should be part of the institution's executive body.

- Find a listening architect.

- Pray for the grace of limitless energy.

- Cancel all other plans for the duration.

- Be endlessly courteous but take no nonsense.

Notes

1. Reports of awards online at:
   http://www-lib.girton.cam.ac.uk/about/RIBA.htm.
   http://www-lib.girton.cam.ac.uk/about/civic.trust.htm.
   http://www-lib.girton.cam.ac.uk/about/SCONUL.htm.
2. C.J. Kitching, *Archive Buildings in the United Kingdom, 1993–2005* (Chichester: Phillimore, 2007), and Alison Wilson and Elmar Mittler, *Furtherance of Academic Excellence: Documentation of New Library Buildings in Cambridge* (Göttingen: Niedersachsische Staats- und Universitätsbibliothek, 2006).

3. Email interview with author, December 2010.
4. Email interview with author, December 2010.
5. Email interview with author, December 2010.
6. Email interview with author, December 2010.
7. Frances Gandy, Client Comment Document, submitted to SCONUL Awards Panel, 2006 (unpublished).

8

Conclusion

Abstract: Can we conclude anything about the new directions in which liaison librarianship may now be going? As the JISC *Libraries of the Future Project* demonstrates, the future of libraries themselves is now up for debate, not just the career trajectories of liaison librarians in particular. A new preoccupation with 'embedded librarianship' has recently emerged as liaison librarians begin to realise that their continued existence may depend not only on remaining visible within the academic community but on convincing that community that the services they offer are critical to the academic research endeavour. There is a drive towards achieving closeness to the research process, and towards integrating the library with research output. All these case studies have demonstrated in their own way this new impulse towards integration and collaboration, and have shown the immense flexibility, adaptability, intelligence and commitment of liaison librarians, which will undoubtedly ensure their long-term survival.

Key words: academic liaison, bibliometrics, embedded librarians, e-Scholarship, faculty liaison, marketing, open access, RAE, REF, scholarly communication, subject librarians, subject specialists, virtual worlds.

The profile of liaison librarianship has changed interestingly in the time it has taken to research the case studies for this book. We have moved into a recession-hit space in which the nature of librarianship and the value of libraries themselves are up for debate. Role-redefinition is in the very air librarians breathe, their willingness to adapt and mould themselves to the requirements of changing times an essential element in their survival tool-kit.

'What is the Library of the Future?' asked the JISC in its high-profile 2009 campaign. In a series of events, printed resources, Web 2.0 services and podcast interviews it provided a platform for much-needed discussion of the issues. Can the academic library retain its traditional place at the heart of campus life? What will be the impact of repositories and open access on the delivery of library resources, and the effect of the digitisation juggernaut on the accessibility of scholarly resources? In a series of three public question and answer debates on 2 April 2009, Sarah Thomas of the Bodleian Library, Robert Darnton of Harvard University Library, Santiago de la Mora of Google Book Search's European partnership, Professor Peter Murray-Rust and Chris Batt OBE worked hard to articulate what libraries meant to them, what services they could deliver, and what people needed them for. They wrestled admirably, too, with the issue of what librarians of the future will actually do. Sarah Thomas said:

> Library buildings will remain at the centre of the university, 'bringing people to explore exhibitions, to house teaching, to provide spaces for study. Libraries will be for collaboration, learning, and creating new knowledge. Staff will expand their skills, but most important will be their ability to collaborate with many partners.[1]

'We must shift from "librarian" to "knowledge warrior" – people committed to wanting to change the relationship between the information and the people who want it,' said Chris Batt. 'The mission needs to be to remove all barriers to access. In terms of public access, we need to forge a universal right to knowledge. That means integrating knowledge into everyday life, and empowering everyone to want to learn.'[2] 'We must digitise and democratise,' said Robert Darnton, recognising the problem that libraries have traditionally been designed to serve just specific constituencies. 'We need to open them up – not by opening physical doors, but through digitisation.'[3]

The changing role of the liaison librarian

Books and articles have gradually begun to appear tackling head-on the conundrum of the liaison librarian's changing role. John W. East's (2007) article, 'The future role of the academic liaison librarian', starts with the grim scenario of the University of Bangor's 2005 decision to make all its subject librarians redundant, and drives in a determinedly upward trajectory through developments since then, showing how liaison librarians' spheres of activity have increased and multiplied, their reinvented selves rising phoenix-like from the ashes of the Bangor tragedy.[4] Information Literacy teaching, virtual reference work, the provision of advanced, subject-related research support, Copyright and Intellectual Property expertise, the management of metadata issues for digital publishing, data curation, assistance with IT issues – liaison librarians have moved resolutely into all these areas and acquitted themselves admirably as the intelligent, adaptable, enthusiastic professionals they are. East's tongue-in-cheek summary of the liaison librarian's new skill set highlights the paradox which is the problem:

> From reading the literature, a composite picture emerges of the liaison librarian of the future. It shows a young,

> outgoing professional who is comfortable hanging out in campus cafes and student halls of residence and able to communicate easily with undergraduate students. At the same time, he or she will be a subject expert, with advanced knowledge of the literature of one or more disciplines and able to work closely with academic staff and postgraduate students. On top of this, our liaison librarian will be extremely proficient with technology and an expert with various software packages used for teaching and research.
>
> Clearly there is nobody who fits this Identikit picture ... We cannot go on pretending that liaison librarians can provide such an impossibly wide range of services.

The point is well worth making: by aspiring to be super-librarians – all things to all readers – we risk losing our credibility.

In 'Scholarly communications: planning for the integration of liaison librarian roles', Joy Kirchner describes a 2009 project at the University of British Columbia Library which aimed to define the Library's role in scholarly communication, and identified liaison librarians as key players in helping to engage with the academic community in this area.[5] It was hoped that the project might clarify how liaison roles could potentially shift to meet new scholarly practices and research behaviour, and could bring liaison librarians closer to the research and faculty research processes on campus. The liaison librarians were asked to conduct an 'environmental scan' of scholarly communications activities in their discipline, using a data-gathering tool adapted from Lee Van Orsdel's *Faculty Activism in Scholarly Communications – Opportunity Assessment Instrument*.[6] In addition, 17 UBC liaison librarians took advantage of the opportunity, by chance available at the same time, to be field librarians in the ARL's study on new publications models. This involved interviewing researchers about how they were engaging with the new models of scholarship, and helped clarify for the librarians how their roles could be usefully expanded to encompass such conversations. All found the experience rewarding, allowing them not only to learn about researchers' specialisms, but also to see first-hand how scholars communicate and keep up to date. For several liaison librarians the conversations resulted in invitations to work with the faculty member to develop a new publishing project – a gratifyingly positive outcome. Health Science liaison librarians found they could focus their skills on facilitating compliance with the new Public Access mandates introduced by the Canadian Institutes of Health research and the US National Institutes of Health (as well as other bodies). Linkages were created between the Library's institutional repository and the University's Office of Research Services systems which made it easy for researchers to deposit their CIHR and NIH grant-funded publications in the repository, following the workflow of the Research Office's grant-funding management system. The Library thus found itself newly visible in the grant application process, and was pleased to find that grant managers in the Research Office were actively encouraging researchers to contact liaison librarians to help strengthen the research component of their grant application. It was recognised, too, that there was potential for useful connections and partnerships between liaison librarians and the University of British Columbia Press, but there was some way to go before these were firmly established. The possibility of providing support for editors who wished to transition their journals to an open access model was being investigated.

Millie Jackson's (2010) study *Subject Specialists in the 21st Century* deals maturely with the 'evolving' nature of the liaison role.[7] While the subject specialist continues to function usefully as an evaluator and recommender of materials, she says, the scope of these materials and the range of the librarian's skills are now significantly broader than in the past. Like Joy Kirchner at UBC, Jackson recognises that the subject specialist must adopt a more consultative and collaborative role with reader–clients, and be active in the advocacy of digital repositories and other e-scholarship resources.

Embedded librarianship

The concept of 'embedded librarianship' begins to feature in the literature from around 2005 onwards, with Barbara I. Dewey's comprehensive survey of new possibilities, 'The embedded librarian: strategic campus collaborations', sounding an imperative call to battle for all librarians wondering what on earth to do next:

> The metaphor of 'embedded librarian' is inspired by the recent phenomenon of embedding journalists into various military sectors during the Iraq war and its aftermath. The concept of embedding implies a more comprehensive integration of one group with another to the extent that the group seeking to integrate is experiencing and observing, as nearly as possible, the daily life of the primary group. Embedding requires more direct and purposeful interaction than acting in parallel with another person, group, or activity. Overt purposefulness makes embedding an appropriate definition of the most comprehensive collaborations for librarians in the higher education community.[8]

Among the various areas in which she proposes the librarian can be usefully embedded – teaching, fundraising, library coffee-shops, the university's website, or virtual space – the research arena is highlighted as appropriate, even essential.

> Integration with scholarly resources is a given for academic research. Research accomplished in partnership with librarians who are subject experts in the appropriate discipline occurs more on an informal basis where librarians are acknowledged as being key to the project or publication's success. Increasing research partnerships in a more formal sense, where librarians are directly contributing to the outcome, requires a deeper level of embeddedness than casual contact. It requires a sophisticated knowledge of faculty research and an ability to determine how one's own expertise, both as a librarian and as subject expert, can contribute.
>
> (ibid., p. 8)

It is towards this 'deeper level of embeddedness' in the research context that liaison librarians are now increasingly aspiring. In his 2007 article, 'Librarians as partners in e-research,' D. Scott Brandt describes how Purdue libraries have been promoting and seeking collaboration between librarians and academics in engineering, science and technology on sponsored research projects.[9] Their outreach has established that researchers have a clear need for the skills librarians can offer in the collection, organisation, description, curation and archiving of data – researchers confirm that they lack time to organise data sets, need help describing data for discovery, want new ways to manage data and need help archiving it. Librarians have therefore been able to involve themselves usefully and relevantly in an impressive range of science and technology projects:

For instance, the libraries are working with one collaborator in analysing water quality data files straight off a sensor (a water logger that records flow, elements in the water, etc.) in the agronomy department. An NIH proposal for a biology resource required having a plan for archiving data, and librarians were asked to be part of the grant. An engineering project sought library science expertise in building metadata for an ontology that allows tracking of data through the workflow. Most recently, a research group working on space exploration came to the libraries to ask if they could 'park their research' with the repository until new funding becomes available. They all view the libraries as 'trusted' partners.

(ibid., p. 366)

Brandt admits that the Purdue experience has been significantly boosted by the fact that Purdue librarians are 'tenure track faculty and are seen as peers on campus' (ibid., p. 367). Without having to engage, as many UK liaison librarians would have to do, in the initial battle to valorise their existence in the academic context, the Purdue library staff have been able to start from a point of important advantage.

Jake Carlson and Ruth Kneale provide a 2011 update on the situation at Purdue in their article, 'Embedded librarianship in the research context: navigating new waters'.[10] They describe Purdue's project-based strategy, through which librarians develop relationships with faculty by identifying their research needs, and by proposing faculty–librarian collaborations to address those needs. The librarians then also help to secure funding to support the collaborations. They accept that becoming an embedded librarian can be a challenging business which can often remove the librarian from his or her comfort zone, and offer a range of advice. They suggest:

Be a team player, as you will need to understand how the whole team works, and be able to play well with others. Secure support from your organization and colleagues, have an entrepreneurial mindset, and be prepared to accept risk. Know how to translate library science to other disciplines, build trusted relationships and above all, 'Don't just think, but act outside of the box!'

(ibid., pp. 168–9)

Models of Embedded Librarianship, the final report of a research project commissioned by the Special Libraries Association between 2007 and 2009, provides endorsement and enthusiastic advocacy of the concept as the major way forward for academic liaison librarians.[11] It accepts that the term 'embedded librarianship' is widely used in the professional literature and describes a variety of services. It covers the work of the academic librarian who participates in an academic course, teaching information literacy skills, as well as the work of librarians in research institutes who are located in offices close to their customer groups rather than in a central library, so that they can work more closely with their customers. It encompasses the role of the medical librarian who goes on 'rounds' and participates in clinical care teams. The criterion for 'embeddedness' for the purposes of the report was 'the provision of specialized services to specific groups', and the authors provide an interesting analysis of the qualifications held by the librarians in their survey. Some 84 per cent of those participating held an ALA- accredited Master's degree in Library or Information Science; 44 per cent also held a bachelor's degree in a field relevant to the clients they served, and 23 per cent held a relevant advanced degree. For this new wave of embedded librarians, the trend is interestingly towards high academic qualifications in a subject area relevant to the customer base – does anyone hear an amused 'Told you so!' from the ghosts of the tried and trusted subject librarians of yesteryear?

For the writers of the 2011 RIN RLUK report *The Value of Libraries for Research and Researchers*, embeddedness is also the Holy Grail of the new Library canon. 'Specialist staff [must] work in partnership with academic departments,' it proclaims in one of its key messages.

> Information specialists – both subject specialists and those with a specific focus on the needs of researchers – form a significant group of the library staff in most institutions. The researchers who make use of them see them as vital. But too often information specialists and researchers are not well connected. Putting that right can alter specialists' roles profoundly, shifting them away from more traditional collection management roles. Where this change has taken place, information specialists take a more proactive role, working in partnership with academic departments and acting as consultants. Such developments have been welcomed by heads of departments and researchers.[12]

The future for academic liaison?

Librarians must cast off the 'invisibility cloaks' which have been the internet's legacy to them, and work hard to reconnect in noticeable, appreciated ways with researchers. If researchers no longer come to the physical library, librarians must find reasons to go them, and to fill the gaps in their knowledge and understanding of researchers' needs. 'Such an approach can lead to a strong service culture permeating the library,' says the report, 'increasing researcher satisfaction, as well as winning recognition and respect for the library across the institution' (ibid., p. 7).

Now, in June 2011, the aspiring liaison librarian may be attracted by the job vacancy advertised by King's College London, whose 'Centre for e-Research is seeking a Research associate with strong technical and software development skills to work on e-research projects'. The post offers the opportunity to contribute to the development of the digital and research infrastructure at Kings, and to explore other e-research possibilities. It will involve working on the Sharing Ancient Wisdoms (SAWS) project, which investigates ways of publishing and interacting with digital collections of manuscripts and texts, especially Greek and Arabic wisdom literature. Candidates are expected to be qualified in information or computer science, or have a humanities degree with a strong technical component. (Graduates of TCD's Digital Arts and Humanities programme or Glasgow's HATII institute come to mind). We have moved startlingly far from the job description of the traditional academic librarian, who may even ten years ago have entered the profession expecting his or her liaison duties to extend no further than talking to students about the mysteries of the classification system, or guiding the elderly professor to where his favourite print bibliographies were kept on the shelf.

Academic liaison in the Arts: a personal view

For me, it has been interesting experiencing at first hand the challenges of developing a professional specialism which is still in many ways a work in progress. 'Alice, your role is evolving!' I was once told by a line manager to whom I had expressed frustration at not knowing exactly what was expected of me in the job. Evolution is rarely a painless process, however. Coming to the post of Academic Liaison Librarian for Arts and Divinity at the start of 2007, I found my own situation fraught with difficulty. I was one of only two liaison librarians at my university, and my colleague and I faced the daunting task of dividing the entire universe of knowledge between us. I assumed responsibility for the 17 departments in the faculties of Arts and Divinity and she took the nine in the faculties of Science and Medicine. I was expected to know as much about the resources for Art History as about the business information needs of economists and management students. I absorbed as much subject knowledge as I could about the disparate areas I now covered, which included Art History, Classics, Economics, English, Film Studies, History, International Relations, Management, Modern Languages, Music, Philosophy and Social Anthropology. Although we were designated 'academic liaison librarians' in the exciting new twenty-first-century terminology, my colleague and I were clearly perceived by the academic world at large as simply 'subject librarians', and were welcomed as such by academic staff.

It was clear from early on that we would have to work hard to define our purpose and to persuade both our academic and our library colleagues that there was more to our liaison roles than that of subject librarian. We had to stress the many other directions in which we planned to develop. With visibility crucial to the role, we created academic liaison web pages explaining our mission and setting out our services. We foregrounded our teaching, emphasising that we would now take this beyond the traditional 'database search techniques' classes and offer new sessions on things like setting up RSS feeds, creating subject portals, 'optimising Google' and using bibliographic referencing services such as RefWorks and

Endnote. The response to this extended programme was enthusiastic and gratifying, and we found ourselves particularly busy with classes at the start of each semester. We also found time to work on additional teaching projects; in my case, developing an interactive online library-skills tutorial to run from the web pages, providing self-help guidance for students and staff on how to satisfy a wide range of information needs, and my colleague worked on developing the potential of Second Life as an environment for information literacy tuition.

We also had to stress the fact that our activities needed to be outward-facing and to take us beyond the Library. We went out to speak to people, making the most of every opportunity to communicate with our Schools and departments, and creating opportunities where none were forthcoming. We addressed School councils and lunchtime seminars, delivered 'staff update sessions' and organised common-room coffee visits. We spoke at staff and student induction days, networked at GRADSkills conferences and inveigled our way into the busy programme of orientation-week activities. We were presenters at an open forum of the Teaching, Learning and Assessment Committee, outlining the purpose of academic liaison and the value of information literacy teaching. Our theme was consistently, 'The Library has much to offer. Tell us what you are doing so that we can match its provision to your needs.' Sometimes our work developed in response to events in the larger academic community. When the year's enhancement theme required that information skills teaching be offered during reading week, we met that demand. When the first-year experience was to be enriched by instruction on how to read electronic books, that need was also met.

While I enjoyed the gentler outward-facing project of setting up the Friends of the Library, described in Chapter 6, with the new 'town and gown' liaison opportunities it offered, I was also excited to be involved in 2007–8 in managing the Library's contribution to the University's RAE submission. Reporting to staff in the RAE Office, I for four months led a team of library assistants who checked and made database entries for each of the publications submitted by the 500 or so St Andrews academic staff. An intensive exercise, it gave me the opportunity to engage with the academic life of the university, discover the research specialisms of staff in all departments, and prove that the librarian's bibliographic skills are integral to any project of this kind.

Establishing the role of Academic Liaison service internally within the Library proved a more intractable challenge. This was a library not ideally prepared for the arrival of its new liaison librarians. Serviced-based, with no tradition of even subject librarians in its long history, the University of St Andrews Library lacked the natural launch-pad for Academic Liaison. A natural evolutionary stage had been bypassed, leaving my colleague and me uncertain from the start of our place in the structure. Our appointments increased the number of professional library staff from seven to nine, and introduced a layer of senior staff which the institution had little previous experience of accommodating. Existing service departments were of necessity already doing parts of the 'inward-facing' elements of our jobs, and we had to work sensitively to reclaim these. Teaching about the use of electronic databases, for example, now became our responsibility, leaving electronic resources staff to continue with the demanding technical and financial aspects of the service. We were expected to engage at some level, too, with collection management, and to work with the Collections Team on this. Defining just how far I was to be involved with this, however, became a difficult issue for me. As I was not working with the collections on a daily basis, lacked the Collections Team's detailed knowledge of the stock and had no line-management connection with them, I found it difficult to make judgements on the various issues referred to me. I felt constantly as though I were being parachuted into situations about which I had little or no background knowledge, and airlifted out again after I had hazarded a hopeful guess at the solution. I was frustrated, too, to find that, since book orders went directly from academic staff to Acquisitions, I was largely unaware of what stock was being ordered, and I came quickly to miss the system with which I had been familiar in other libraries where book orders were sent to the subject librarians for initial processing. Though I was billed as 'first point of contact between Schools and the Library', I found in practice that I often was not. Academics continued to go directly to the Collections Team about collections issues and to the Acquisitions Team with purchasing enquiries, bypassing me altogether.

It was difficult at times to avoid the depressing thought that Academic Liaison might perhaps have arrived just too late for this library. It seemed, indeed, as though Liaison had simply been grafted onto a staff structure which had not changed to accommodate it. Although staff on all sides largely dealt with the situation with good will and good humour, it was clear to everyone that there was frequently a lack of clarity about who was responsible for what, and that duplication of effort and general confusion were at times the unintended and unfortunate consequences of the creation of these new posts. Were we pushing against the grain in trying to establish this new area of service, I found myself wondering? Was Academic Liaison really the way to go?

Now, nearly five years on, things have changed substantially for the better. My colleague and I have 'hung in there' and in

2011 are pleased and relieved to be part of an expanded and recently restructured Academic Liaison Team which allows us to function with increased effectiveness and confidence. We have a new Social Sciences Liaison Librarian; responsibility for the Institutional Repository now lies within Liaison, which incorporates its staff; we supervise the two library assistants who work on our electronic reading lists project; significant efforts by senior managers have resulted in new work flows which ensure that all subject-related enquiries reach Liaison staff as appropriate. The goal of being the established and recognisable 'first points of contact' for our readers seems at last to be achievable and in reach. Helpful, too, has been our inclusion in regular meetings of the Collections Advisory Group and the Strategic Management Group, which have kept us informed about collections and other issues about which we need to know in order to fulfil our liaison roles.

My own liaison post now seems to be evolving into a hopeful, more coherent new shape. The team as a whole is about to assume more research–specific responsibilities, and I have myself recently been tasked with seeking out Digital Humanities projects in my subject areas with which I might provide support. I will turn with enthusiasm in this exciting new direction.

My five years in post have shown me that introducing Academic Liaison to a library alters it fundamentally. The focus of the library's activities changes. Its services must be seen as radiating *from* Academic Liaison, the team itself as central and crucial to the library's mission. Academic Liaison can only survive if it is integrated and at the heart of the library's ethos. Liaison librarians need to remain unfazed by the uncertainty of the library landscapes in which they operate, and by the fluidity of their roles as they develop. They should be alert to the opportunities the situation offers, embrace change and be vocal and confident about claiming centre stage for themselves.

Case study round-up

The liaison projects highlighted in our case studies are all interesting products of these changing and uncertain times, and the librarians involved in them have all wrestled in their individual ways with the need to seek out areas of usefulness in which to apply their many skills. Vicki Cormie has thought most excitingly 'out of the box', as the Purdue librarians advise, and has seized opportunities which have taken her technical and medical collection building expertise to the Malawi library where they were much needed. She was in a real way 'embedded' in the close-knit team of academics and administrators donating their support to the project, and found herself able to contribute in important ways to the mission as a whole. My own experience of setting up the Friends of the Library and organising our King James Library Lectures again illustrates that not all liaison ventures need to be electronic or web-based. The opportunity to establish new networks of library supporters has been useful and interesting, and has noticeably increased the Library's visibility in both town and gown communities. I feel I have, as Robert Darnton exhorts in the Libraries of the Future Debate, helped to 'open up' the Library to a constituency which would normally be 'outside looking in', and have raised its profile as a cultural space where books are not just stored but the ideas inside them discussed with intelligence. Again, Frances Gandy's library building experience at Girton is a perfect example of a librarian embedded in a project, collaborating in real ways with academics, architects, administrators, fundraisers and other librarians to bring a building project to splendid fruition. She brought to the team her expert specialist knowledge of how a library should look and work, and had the stressful pleasure of guiding the team members towards making her vision a reality.

Susan Ashworth at Glasgow University has been one of an increasing number of librarians to cross the boundary between books and bibliometrics and to have embedded herself and her team in the library-related, but still essentially administrative, Research Office sphere of activity where the librarian's skills are used to collect, correct and collate. Liaison skills have proved newly useful in this exercise where accurate publication details have had to be elicited from busy academics, and, while the RAE has been a uniquely British venture, parallel projects in Europe and elsewhere (e.g. the Netherlands' Standard Evaluation Protocol and Australia's Research Quality Framework) indicate that library involvement is likely soon to be accepted as the desired norm in these places also.

Other boundaries have been crossed by Robin Ashford in Portland, Oregon, who moved enthusiastically into the virtual world of Second Life, becoming the much-needed embedded librarian who helped orientate new students venturing in there, and guided them towards acquiring appropriate information literacy skills. Her work with faculty in this context has clearly contributed significantly to the success of the project, her position as adjunct instructor on the courses she was involved with testifying to her close collaboration with academic staff, and her full integration into the team.

Liaisons between the library and the digital publishing worlds have also, as we have seen, been fruitful new directions for some. While there are variations in scale between, for example, the vast California Digital Library venture and the more niche Glasgow Emblem Digitisation Project, it is clear that digital publishing is the future for scholarship, and that there is a place in that arena for librarians' new skills, though they may have to elbow their way in. Trinity College Dublin's Digital Humanities Degree and Glasgow University's Humanities and Technical Innovation Institute look to be producing useful graduates with their sights trained on this area, and the fact that HATII's Information Management & Preservation Master's degree is CILIP accredited should be seen as significant. Meanwhile, far-sighted institutional repository workers such as Jackie Proven at St Andrews continue to do important new liaison work with converts in the academic community, encouraging them to use increasingly popular Open Access models for the publication of both books and journals, and working collaboratively with them to host attractive, efficiently accessible publications alongside their repository platforms.

Do all these projects hint at a degree of desperation in the world of liaison librarianship as we rack our brains for something – anything – we can do next, now that Google does most of our old jobs for us? Are we like Stephen Leacock's hero 'riding madly off in all directions' or heading purposefully in a carefully chosen few?[13] Presumably only time will tell. If some of the directions we have tried to push in now turn out eventually to be dead ends, we will be able to look back on this period of pushing the boundaries as simply a useful but necessary experiment.

Reports of the death of the book are greatly exaggerated, as Sarah Thomas said at the JISC *Future of the Libraries* debate in October 2009.[14] So too, we can hope, are those of the death of the liaison librarian. The liaison librarian is, after all, surely the most infinitely enduring, resilient, adaptable, ingenious, persistent, imaginative, long-suffering professional specimen the information world can possibly offer. If these case studies have done nothing else, they have shown liaison librarians to be inveterate shape-shifters, as Darwinianly capable of feeding neat bibliographic details into a database as of throwing up a new library building when one is required. It will take more than a few Google searches to wipe them out.

Notes

1. JISC Libraries of the Future. Blog for the JISC Campaign, Session 1, 2 April 2009. Available at: *http://librariesofthefuture. jiscinvolve.org/wp/2009/04/02/libraries-of-the-future-session–1/*.
2. Ibid.
3. JISC Libraries of the Future brochure (2009). Available at: *http://www.jisc.ac.uk/media/documents/publications/lotfbrochure.pdf*.
4. John W. East, 'The future role of the academic liaison librarian: a literature review', *E-Prints in Library and Information Science* (2007). Available at: *http://eprints.rclis.org/handle/10760/10561*.
5. Joy Kirchner, 'Scholarly communications: planning for the integration of liaison librarian roles', *Research Library Issues: A Bimonthly Report from ARL, CNI, and SPARC*, 265 (August 2009): 22–8. Available at: *http://www.arl.org/resources/pubs/rli/archive/rli265.shtml*.
6. Lee Van Orsdel, *Faculty Activism in Scholarly Communications – Opportunity Assessment Instrument*. Tool developed for the ACRL/ARL Institute for Scholarly Communications. Available at: *www.arl.org/bm~doc/opp.pdf*.
7. Millie Jackson, *Subject Specialists in the 21st Century* (Oxford: Chandos, 2010).
8. Barbara I. Dewey, 'The embedded librarian', *Resource Sharing & Information Networks* 17(1) (2005): 6.
9. D. Scott Brandt, 'Librarians as partners in e-research: Purdue university libraries promote collaboration', *C&RL News* (June 2007): 365–9.
10. Jake Carlson and Ruth Kneale, 'Embedded librarianship in the research context: navigating new waters', *C&RL News* (March 2011): 167–70.

11. David Shumaker and Mary Talley, *Models of Embedded Librarianship: Final Report* (2009). Available at: *http://www.sla.org/pdfs/EmbeddedLibrarianshipFinalRptRev.pdf*.

12. RIN/RLUK, *The Value of Libraries for Research and Researchers* (March 2011). Available at: *http://www.rluk.ac.uk/content/value-libraries-research-and-researchers*.

13. 'Lord Ronald . . . flung himself upon his horse and rode madly off in all directions.' Stephen Leacock, 'Gertrude the Governess', in *Nonsense Novels* (New York: John Lane, 1911).

14. JISC Libraries of the Future. Blog for the JISC Campaign, Session 1, 2 April 2009. Available at: *http://librariesofthefuture.jiscinvolve.org/wp/2009/04/02/libraries-of-the-future-session-1/*.

References and further reading

Adams, Alison, Rawles, Stephen and Saunders, Alison (1999) *A Bibliography of French Emblem Books of the Sixteenth and Seventeenth Centuries*, Geneva: Librairie Droz.

Ashford, Robin, Headley, S. and Zijdemans-Boudreau, A. (2009a) 'Do educators need a Second Life? Exploring possibilities for technology-based distance learning in higher education', in I. Gibson et al. (eds) *Proceedings of Society for Information Technology & Teacher Education International Conference*, Chesapeake, VA: AACE, pp. 1617–22. Available at: *http://www.editlib.org/p/30846*.

Ashford, Robin, Headley, S. and Zijdemans-Boudreau, A. (2009b) 'Faculty preparation for teaching and learning in Second Life', in T. Bastiaens et al. (eds) *Proceedings of World Conference on E-Learning in Corporate, Government, Healthcare, and Higher Education*, Chesapeake, VA: AACE, pp. 2366–8. Available at: *http://www.editlib. org/p/32814*.

Ashford, Robin, Headley, S. and Zijdemans-Boudreau, A. (2009c) 'Immersive virtual worlds in educational practice: introducing educators to Second Life', in T. Bastaiens et al. (eds) *Proceedings of World Conference on E-Learning in Corporate, Government, Healthcare, and Higher Education*, Chesapeake, VA: AACE, pp. 2076–81. Available at: *http://www.editlib.org/p/32770*.

Ashworth, Susan (2009) 'Research support at the University of Glasgow Library', *SCONUL Focus*, 45: 50–1. Available at: *http://www.sconul.ac.uk/publications/newsletter/45/15.pdf*.

Bourg, Chris, Coleman, Ross and Erway, Ricky (2009) *Support for the Research Process: An Academic Library Manifesto. Report Produced by OCLC Research.* Available at: *http://www.oclc.org/research/publications/library/2009/2009-07.pdf*.

Brandt, D. Scott (2007) 'Librarians as partners in e-research: Purdue University Libraries promote collaboration', *C&RL News*, June: 365–9.

Brewerton, Antony (2009) 'Editorial', The Subject Librarian Issue, *SCONUL Focus*, 45: 3–4.

Brown, Laura, Griffiths, Rebecca and Rascoff, Matthew (2007) *University Publishing in a Digital Age: Ithaka Report*, 26 July. Available at: *http://www.arl.org/bm~doc/arl-br-252-253-ithaka.pdf*.

Brownlee, Rowan (2009) 'Research data and repository metadata – policy and technical issues', *Cataloguing & Classification Quarterly*, 47(3/4). Available at: *http://hdl.handle.net/2123/4996*.

Bulger, Monica et al. (2011) *Reinventing Research? Information Practices in the Humanities: A Research Information Network Report*, London: RIN. Available at: *http://www.rin.ac.uk/our-work/using-and-accessing-information-resources/information-use-case-studies-humanities*.

Carlson, Jake and Kneale, Ruth (2011) 'Embedded librarianship in the research context: navigating new waters', *C&RL News*, March: 167–70.

Case, Mary M. and John, Nancy R. (2007) 'Publishing journals @ UIC', *ARL*, 252/253 (June/August). Available at: *http://www.arl.org/bm~doc/arl-br-252-253-uic.pdf*.

Christensen, Sten (2009) 'Sydney eScholarship Repository: a case study', *Educause Australasia Conference*, Perth,

Western Australia, 3–6 May 2009. Paper No. 99.00 EDUCAUSE. Available at: *http://hdl.handle.net/2123/5027*.

Cole, Creagh (1997) 'Electronic texts at the University of Sydney Library'. Available at: *http://www.ariadne.ac.uk/issue8/scholarly-electronic/*.

Cole, Creagh (1999) 'A new continent into literature: the Australian Literature Database at the University of Sydney Library', in *Electronic Publishing '99: Redefining the Information Chain – New Ways and Voices. Proceedings of an ICCC/IFIP Conference Held at the University of Karlskrona/Ronneby, Sweden, 10–12 May, 1999. Paper 9909*, Washington, DC: ICCC Press. Available at: *http://elpub.scix.net/cgi-bin/works/Show?9909*.

Cole, Creagh (n.d.) 'Form and content: historical and literary texts on the World Wide Web at SETIS', available at: *http://www.jcu.edu.au/aff/history/articles/cole.htm*.

Coleman, Ross (2006) 'Field, file, data, conference: towards new modes of scholarly publication', *Sustainable Data from Digital Fieldwork: Proceedings of the Conference held at the University of Sydney, December 2006*. Available at: *http://hdl.handle.net/2123/1300*.

Coleman, Ross (2008) 'Scholarly publishing within an e-scholarship framework – Sydney eScholarship as a model of integration and sustainability', *Open Scholarship: Authority, Community and Sustainability in the Age of Web 2.0, ElPub 2008, 12th International Conference on Electronic Publishing*, Toronto, Canada, June 2008. Available at: *http://hdl.handle.net/2123/1300*.

Coleman, Ross (2009) 'Publishing and the digital library – adding value to scholarship and innovation to business', *Learned Publishing*, 22(4):297–303. doi:10.1087/20090406.

College of DuPage Newsroom (2009) 'College uses Second Life to educate students', 16 November. Available at: *http://*

triblocal.com/glen-ellyn/community/stories/2009/11/college-uses-second-life-to-educate-students/.

Dale, Penny, Holland, Matt and Matthews, Marian (2006) *Subject Librarians: Engaging with the Learning and Teaching Environment*, Aldershot: Ashgate.

Dewey, Barbara I. (2005) 'The embedded librarian', *Resource Sharing & Information Networks*, 17(1): 5–17.

East, John W. (2007) 'The future role of the academic liaison librarian: a literature review', *E-Prints in Library and Information Science*. Available at: *http://eprints.rclis.org/handle/10760/10561*.

Fairbairn, Linden and Rodwell, John (2008) 'Dangerous liaisons? Defining the faculty liaison librarian service model, its effectiveness and sustainability', *Library Management* 29(1/2): 116–24. doi: 10.1108/01435120810844694.

Gaston, Richard (2001) 'The changing role of the subject librarian, with a particular focus on UK developments, examined through a review of the literature', *New Review of Academic Librarianship*, 7(1): 19–36.

Greenhill, Kathryn (2008) 'Do we remove all the walls? Second Life librarianship', Librariesinteract.info, 2008. Available at: *http://researchrepository.murdoch.edu.au/623/1/Published_Version.pdf*.

Greig, Morag (2009) 'Achieving an "Enlightened" publications policy at the University of Glasgow', *Serials*, 22(1): 7–11. Available at: *http:/dx.doi.org/10/1629/227*.

Greig, Morag and Nixon, William (2007) 'On the road to Enlighten-ment: establishing an institutional repository service for the University of Glasgow', *OCLC Systems & Services: International Digital Library Perspectives*, 23(3): 297–309. Available at: *http://dx.doi.org/10.1108/10650750710776431*.

Hahn, Karla L. (2008) *Research Library Publishing Services: New Options for University Publishing*, Washington, DC:

Association of Research Libraries. Available at: *http://www. arl.org/bm~doc/research-library-publishing-services.pdf.*

Hay, Fred J. (1990) 'The subject specialist in the academic library: a review article', *The Journal of Academic Librarianship*, 16(1): 11–17.

Hudson, Rob (2008) 'A little grafting of Second Life into a legal research class', *LLRX.com*, 9 May 2008. Available at: *http://www.llrx.com/features/secondlife.htm.*

Jackson, Millie (2010) *Subject Specialists in the 21st Century*, Oxford: Chandos.

James, Ann-Marie (2008) 'Dotting the DOIs and crossing the ESSNs: librarians' support for the RAE 2008', *Serials*, 21(3): 174–7. Available at: *http://dx.doi.org/10.1629/21174.*

JISC Libraries of the Future (2009a) Blog for the JISC Campaign, Session 1, 2 April, 2009. Available at: *http://librariesofthe future.jiscinvolve.org/wp/2009/04/02/libraries-of-the-future-session-1/.*

JISC Libraries of the Future (2009b) brochure. Available at: *http://www.jisc.ac.uk/media/documents/publications/ lotfbrochure.pdf.*

Key Perspectives Ltd. (2009) *A Comparative Review of Research Assessment Regimes in Five Countries and the Role of Libraries in the Research Assessment Process.* Report commissioned by OCLC Research. Available at: *http://www.oclc.org/research/publications/library/2009/ 2009-09.pdf.*

Kinnie, Jim (2006) 'The embedded librarian: bringing library services to distance learners', in *22nd Annual Conference on Distance Teaching and Learning.* Available at: *http:// www.uwex.edu/disted/conference/Resource_Library/ proceedings/06_4327.pdf.*

Kirchner, Joy (2009) 'Scholarly communications: planning for the integration of liaison librarian roles', *Research Library Issues: A Bimonthly Report from ARL, CNI, and*

SPARC, 265 (August 2009): 22–8. Available at: *http://www.arl.org/resources/pubs/rli/archive/rli265.shtml.*

Kitching, C.J. (2007) *Archive Buildings in the United Kingdom, 1993–2005*, Chichester: Phillimore.

Kosavic, Andrea (2010) 'The York Digital Journals Project: strategies for institutional open journal systems implementations', *College and Research Libraries*, 71 (2010): 310–21. Available at: *http://crl.acrl.org/content/71/4/310.abstract.*

Law, Derek (1999) 'The organization of collection management in academic libraries', in Clare Jenkins and Mary Morley (eds) *Collection Management in Academic Libraries*, 2nd edn, Aldershot: Gower, pp. 15–37.

Lund, Peter and Young, Helen (2007) *Benchmarking Survey of Research Support Provided by 1994 Group Libraries*, Loughborough: University Library.

MacColl, John (2010) *Research Assessment and the Role of the Library.* Report produced by OCLC Research, 2010. Available at: *http://www.oclc.org/research/publications/library/2010/2010-01.pdf.*

Maron, Nancy L. and Smith, K. Kirby (2008) *Current Models of Digital Scholarly Communication: Results of an Investigation Conducted by Ithaka for the Association of Research Libraries*, Washington, DC: ARL. Available at: *http://www.arl.org/bm~doc/current-models-report.pdf.*

Martin, J.V. (1996) 'Subject specialization in British University Libraries: a second survey', *Journal of Librarianship and Information Science*, 28(3): 159–69.

Nesson, Rebecca and Nesson, Charles (2008) 'The case for education in virtual worlds', *Space and Culture*, 11(3): 273–84. Available at: *http://sac.sagepub.com/content/11/3/273.short.*

Pinfield, Stephen C. (2001) 'The changing role of subject librarians in academic libraries', *Journal of Librarianship and Information Science*, 33(1): 32–8.

Proven, Jackie and Aucock, Janet (2011) 'Increasing uptake at St Andrews – strategies for developing the research repository', *ALISS Quarterly*, 6(3): 6–9. Special issue: Library Services for the 21st Century.

Rawles, Stephen (n.d.) 'A spine of information headings for emblem-related electronic resources', in Mara R. Wade, *Digital Collections and the Management of Knowledge: Renaissance Emblem Literature as a Case Study for the Digitization of Rare Texts and Images*. Available at: *http://www.digicult.info/downloads/dc_emblemsbook_lowres.pdf*.

Research Information Network (2007) *Researchers' Use of Academic Libraries and their Services*, RIN Report (2007). *http://www.rin.ac.uk/our-work/using-and-accessing-information-resources/researchers-use-academic-libraries-and-their-services*.

Research Information Network (2008) *Ensuring a Bright Future for Research Libraries: A Guide for Vice-Chancellors and Senior Institutional Managers*. RIN Report (2008). Available at: *http://www.rin.ac.uk/our-work/using-and-accessing-information-resources/ensuring-bright-future-research-libraries*.

Research Information Network (2011) *The Value of Libraries for Research and Researchers: RIN/ RLUK Report* (March). Available at: *http://www.rluk.ac.uk/content/value-libraries-research-and-researchers*.

Robinson-Garcia, Nicolas and Torres-Salinas, Daniel (2011) 'Librarians "embedded" in research', *CILIP Update*, (June): 44–6.

Rodwell, John (2001) 'Dinosaur or dynamo? The future for the subject specialist reference librarian', *New Library World*, 102(1/2): 48–52.

Schiff, Lisa (2009) 'Creating the Mark Twain Project Online', *Learned Publishing*, 22: 191–8. Available at: *http://escholarship.org/uc/item/7xt0z56t*.

Shapiro, Lorna (2005) *Establishing and Publishing an Online Peer-review Journal: Action Plan, Resourcing and Costs* (OJS Project Report, 2005). Available at: *http://pkp. sfu.ca/files/OJS_Project_Report_Shapiro.pdf.*

Shumaker, David and Talley, Mary (2009) *Models of Embedded Librarianship: Final Report.* Available at: *http://www.sla. org/pdfs/EmbeddedLibrarianshipFinalRptRev.pdf.*

Smith, Jacqueline (2010) Interview with Christine Madsen, in 'Buried treasure', *Floreat Domus, Balliol College News,* 16: 46.

Toon, James (forthcoming) *Supporting Research Dissemination: Project Report,* forthcoming from OCLC. Available at: *http://www.oclc.org/research/activities/desirability/default .htm.*

Wade, Mara R. (2004) *Digital Collections and the Management of Knowledge: Renaissance Emblem Literature as a Case Study for the Digitization of Rare Texts and Images* (DigiCULT, 2004). Available at: *http://www.digicult.info/ downloads/dc_emblemsbook_lowres.pdf.*

Walters, T. O. (2007) 'Reinventing the library: how repositories are causing librarians to rethink their professional roles', *Portal: Libraries and the Academy,* 7(2): 213–25. Available at: *http://smartech.gatech.edu/handle/1853/14421.*

Williams, Karen and Jaguscewski, Janice (2011) *Transforming Liaison Roles.* Forthcoming Report in the ARL's *New Roles for New Times Series.* Available at: *http://www.arl. org/rtl/plan/nrnt/nrntliaison.shtml.*

Wilson, Alison and Mittler, Elmar (2006) *Furtherance of Academic Excellence: Documentation of New Library Buildings in Cambridge,* Göttingen: Niedersachsische Staats-und Universitätsbibliothek.

Wusteman, Judith (2008) 'Virtual research environments: what is the librarian's role?' (Editorial) *JOLIS,* 40(2): 67–70.

Websites

Friends of St Andrews University Library website *http:// www.st-andrews.ac.uk/library/friends/*.

Girton College, Cambridge: Reports of architectural awards: *http://www-lib.girton.cam.ac.uk/about/RIBA.htm.* *http://www-lib.girton.cam.ac.uk/about/SCONUL.htm.* *http://www-lib.girton.cam.ac.uk/about/civic_trust.htm.*

JISC Enrich – Enhancement Strand. *Overview of University of Glasgow's Enlighten project. http://www.jisc.ac.uk/ whatwedo/programmes/inf11/sue2/enrich.*

King James Library Lectures website *http://www.st-andrews. ac.uk/library/news/lectures/*.

PKP (Public Knowledge Project) *The Division of Labor on a Campus Hosting Open Journal Systems and Open Conference Systems.* PowerPoint presentation from PKP. Available at: *http://pkp.sfu.ca/files/Division%20of%20 Labor.pdf.*

SURF Copyright Toolbox. Available at: *http://copyrighttool box.surf.nl/copyrighttoolbox/.*

Van Orsdel, Lee *Faculty Activism in Scholarly Communications – Opportunity Assessment Instrument.* Tool developed for the ACRL/ARL Institute for Scholarly Communications. Available at: *www.arl.org/bm~doc/opp.pdf.*

Vicki's Adventures in Malawi, *http://vickimalawi.blogspot. com/.*

Presentations and Flickrsets by Robin Ashford

An Academic Librarian in Second Life, http://www.slideshare. net/RobinAshford/academic-librarian-in-second-life-presentation.

Blogger profile, *http://www.blogger.com/profile/048670353 52518158417.*

A Consumer Health Librarian's National Library of Medicine Funded Project in Second Life, http://www.slideshare.net/ RobinAshford/consumer-health-librarianinsecondlifefinal.

How Doctors, Nurses, Allied Health Professionals and Patients use Second Life, http://www.slideshare.net/RobinAshford/ how-doctors-nurses-allied-health-professionals-and-patients.

Informal Adult Learning in Second Life, http://www. slideshare.net/RobinAshford/informal-adult-learning-in-second-life.

Robin Ashford's Librarian by Design Blog, *http:// librarianbydesign.blogspot.com/.*

Robin Ashford's Posterous Blog, *http://robinashford.posterous .com/.*

Slides of EDFL675 in Second Life, *http://www.flickr.com/ photos/25095603@N07/sets/72157606936878733/.*

Slides of EDFL625 in Second Life, *http://www.flickr.com/ photos/25095603@N07/sets/72157614072305900/.*

Slides of MLDR550 in Second Life, *http://www.flickr.com/ photos/25095603@N07/sets/72157625447837867/.*

Index

CPSIA information can be obtained at www.ICGtesting.com
Printed in the USA
LVOW102058150513

333803LV00002B/12/P

9 781843 345695